Understanding Medical Immunology

Second Edition

Evelyne M. Kirkwood
Catriona J. Lewis

*Department of Bacteriology and Immunology,
Western Infirmary,
Glasgow,
G11 6NT*

A Wiley Medical Publication

JOHN WILEY & SONS
Chichester · New York · Brisbane · Toronto · Singapore

British Library Cataloguing in Publication Data:
Data available
0 471 91577 7

Library of Congress Cataloging in Publication Data:
Kirkwood, Evelyne M.
  Understanding medical immunology.

  (A Wiley medical publication)
  Includes index.
  1. Immunologic diseases.   2.   Immunology.
I. Lewis, Catriona J.   II. Title.   III. Series.
[DNLM: 1.   Allergy and Immunology. QW 504 K59u]
RC582.K57   1989   616.07′9   87–31747
ISBN 0 471 91577 7

Typeset by Photo graphics, Honiton, Devon
Printed and bound by the Bath Press, Bath, Avon

To our children,

*Martin, Carolyn, David,
and Heather*

and since the last edition, Neil

Contents

Section A **Basic principles**

Section B **Clinical conditions involving immunological mechanisms**

Section C AIDS—acquired immunodeficiency syndrome

Section D Immunological investigation and procedures

Preface

This is not a book for would-be immunologists. It is intended rather for nursing and laboratory staff who are expected to study a little immunology during the course of their training. It may also be useful to some 'mature' members of the medical staff who qualified before immunology featured in the medical curriculum and who have never quite found time to come to terms with the subject.

It is hoped that the free use of diagrams results in a book that is quickly and easily read but at the same time brings out most of the basic immunological concepts.

Preface to the second edition

The welcome success of our first edition of *Understanding Medical Immunology* has prompted us, at the request of our publishers, to introduce a second updated edition on this subject.

Since our first edition was published, there have been considerable advances made in immunological theory and technology which we have tried to cover. The style and structure of the first edition have been maintained but a whole new section on AIDS has been included which we hope will be useful.

Acknowledgements

We are much indebted to Professor Heather Dick, Miss Jean Murdoch, and Miss Margaret Henderson for their helpful advice and would like to thank our publishers John Wiley and Sons for their patience, assistance, and invaluable guidance throughout the preparation of this book. Lastly, but by no means least, we would like to thank our families for their forbearance throughout.

Section A
Basic principles

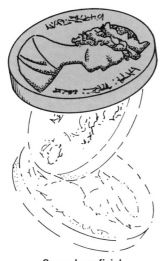

**Some beneficial
effects of the immune system**

Protection against bacterial,
viral, fungal, and parasitic disease

Protection against tumours

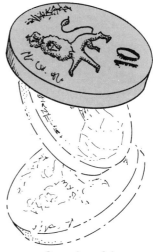

**Some harmful
effects of the immune system**

Conditions such as: Pernicious anaemia
Rheumatoid arthritis
Glomerulonephritis
Asthma
Penicillin allergy
Some types of dermatitis

1. Clinical immunology—some perspectives

Strangely, immunology can be regarded as one of the youngest or one of the oldest, one of the smallest or one of the largest, one of the simplest or one of the most complicated of the medical specialties depending on one's point of view.

Until a few decades ago immunology was closely intermingled and almost synonymous with the specialties that we now know as infectious diseases and microbiology. The main purpose of our immune system is to protect us from infection in its various forms, and one of the greatest discoveries in medicine, immunization, was put into use and saved millions of lives a century and a half before there was any real scientific understanding of the mechanisms involved. But the immune system is a coin with two sides. For a few people, when the coin spins it falls on the unfavourable side, and then, instead of functioning purely as a protective mechanism, immune reactions harmful to the host are produced. It was only when we became aware of some of these harmful mechanisms, in relatively recent times, that immunology separated from the specialty of infectious diseases.

It is generally considered that the subject known as clinical immunology, at least in Britain at the present time, is concerned with the laboratory investigation of patients with immunological problems. This is really only one aspect of a much larger 'parent' specialty concerned with (A) the study of *antigens*★, (B) the diseases caused by antigens, and (C) the management and prevention of these diseases. Because damaging immune reactions can involve

any of the systems of the body, immunology has spread its roots into most branches of medicine. As a result of these ramifications, clinical immunology in its widest sense has not enjoyed any real independence. It is, nevertheless, a major medical specialty.

In addition to dealing with the harmful conditions resulting from activity of the immune system, clinicians and nursing staff are now more involved than ever before in caring for patients who have greatly diminished immune function. This until recently was almost always the result of suppression of the immune response secondary to potent anti-tumour therapy or in the prevention of graft rejection in transplant patients. Indeed, such immune deficiencies can be regarded as a consequence of some of medicine's most powerful modern therapies.

In the early 1980s a new type of secondary immune deficiency was recognized. This followed a new pattern. Firstly, it was not a side effect of medical intervention, and secondly it affected previously healthy individuals. Within a short time a virus was identified as the agent responsible for the condition now known worldwide as AIDS. In this condition the virus infects cells which are an important part of the immune system—hence the development of severe immune deficiency.

Clearly therefore, an understanding of immunology leads to a wider appreciation of the problems experienced by large groups of patients and hopefully in the future to improved management and perhaps complete prevention of their condition.

★ An *antigen* is a foreign substance, usually a protein, which is capable of stimulating the body's immune system.

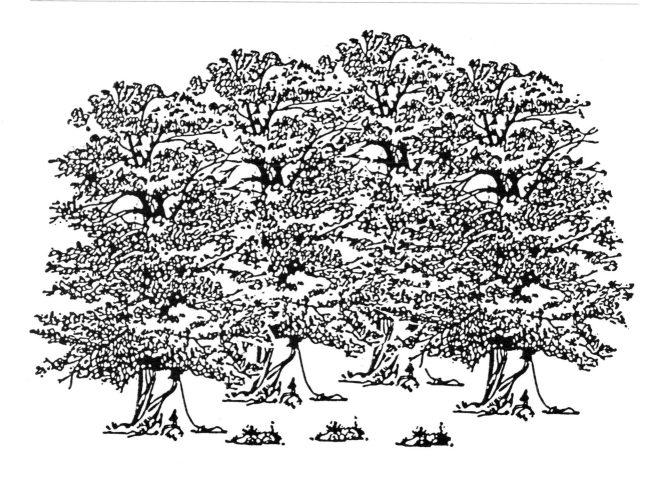

2. A simple or a complicated subject?

In immunology, one very often 'can't see the wood for the trees'. The trees often take the form of jargon, complicated terminology, and abbreviations and obscure the fact that the wood itself is a delightful place to be. Immunology is, in fact, a subject of simple, logical concepts. If one understands these concepts, the jargon presents no problem since it only represents man's cumbersome way of expressing himself.

It is now necessary to introduce some terminology which will gradually become familiar as you read further.

The non-specific path

This path is the first and perhaps the most important leading to that section of the wood concerned with the body's first line of defence against infection. The following are all examples of non-specific defence mechanisms.

Protective mechanical mechanisms, e.g. coughing, sneezing, wafting of the cilia lining the trachea and bronchi.

The presence of substances in secretions which help destroy bacteria, e.g. hydrochloric acid in the stomach, wax in the ears, enzymes in tears.

Cells capable of destroying foreign material as soon as it enters the body, e.g. circulating white blood cells such as *neutrophils*, tissue *macrophages*.

Circulating substances, e.g. a group of substances known collectively as *complement* (to be considered later), a substance known as *interferon* which is important in the prevention of viral infections.

The specific immune path

This path is concerned with the recognition of certain foreign material known as *antigens* and how the immune system can be stimulated to make a very specific immune response leading to their destruc-

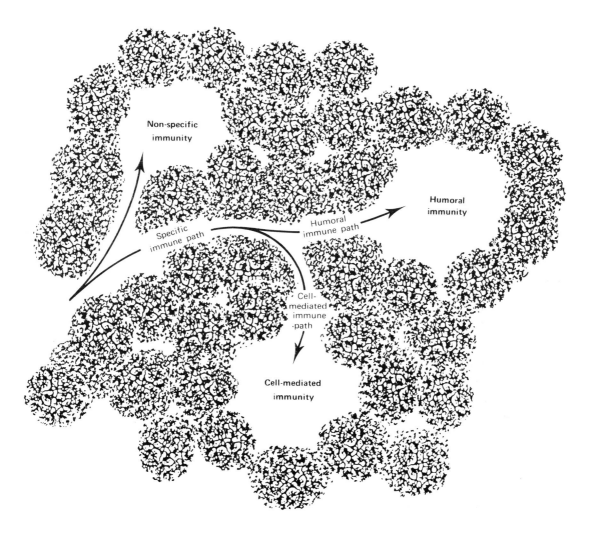

tion. This path branches into the *humoral system* and the *cell-mediated system*.

The humoral system

The humoral system is concerned with the production of circulating proteins known as *immunoglobulins* or *antibodies*. The cells of the humoral system are *B lymphocytes* which, under certain circumstances, become *plasma cells*. It is the plasma cells that produce and release immunoglobulins into the circulation.

B lymphocytes and *plasma cells* are important in the prevention of many *bacterial infections*.

The cell-mediated system

This system is concerned with the activity of cells known as *T lymphocytes* which are capable of specifically destroying *antigenic material* (e.g. foreign material such as microorganisms) which is either fixed in the tissues or inside cells.

T lymphocytes are important in the prevention of many *viral infections*.

The communicating lanes of the immune system

Although it is convenient initially to consider the paths of the immune system as completely separate, there are in fact many lanes leading from one part of the wood to another. As will be seen later, there is considerable interaction between the different sections of the immune system. For example: (1) the specific immune system makes use of cells and chemicals that are important in the non-specific immune system; and (2) cells of the cell-mediated system can greatly influence the type of response produced by the humoral system.

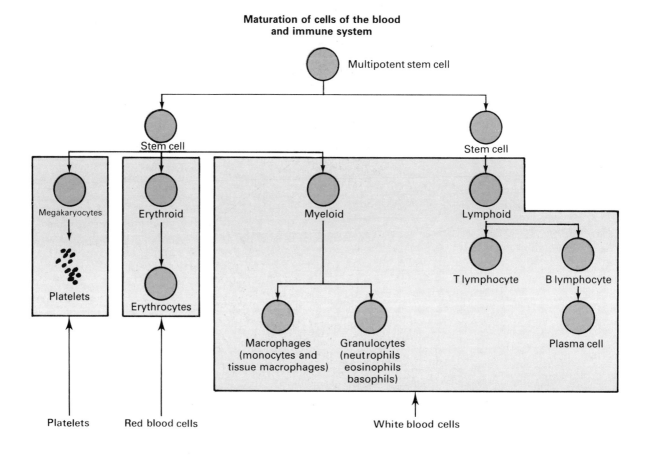

Maturation of cells of the blood and immune system

Multipotent stem cell

Stem cell

Stem cell

Megakaryocytes

Erythroid

Myeloid

Lymphoid

Platelets

Erythrocytes

T lymphocyte

B lymphocyte

Macrophages (monocytes and tissue macrophages)

Granulocytes (neutrophils eosinophils basophils)

Plasma cell

Platelets

Red blood cells

White blood cells

3. Cells of the immune system

The human immune system comprises a variety of cells distributed throughout the body. They are found in the spleen, thymus, lymph nodes, blood, and lymph, and in the respiratory, gastrointestinal, and genitourinary tracts.

These cells can be classified according to function into the following groups:

A. *Cells mainly involved in non-specific immunity*

Phagocytic cells	Mononuclear phagocytes
	Polymorphonuclear phagocytes (neutrophils)
	Eosinophils
Mediator cells	Basophils and mast cells
	Platelets

B. *Cells mainly involved in specific immunity*

Lymphocytes
Plasma cells

The *origins* of all these cell types are stem cells found in the bone marrow. These self-replicating cells differentiate into two types of 'committed' stem cells. One group of stem cells eventually differentiates further and matures to become *platelets, erythrocytes* (*red blood cells*), *monocytes*, or *granulocytes*. The second group produces cells of the *lymphoid line* only.

(It is presumed that the reader has a little knowledge of haematology. It might be helpful to revise the cells of the blood at this stage.)

The mononuclear phagocytes

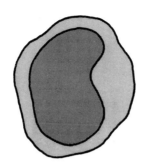

Blood monocyte

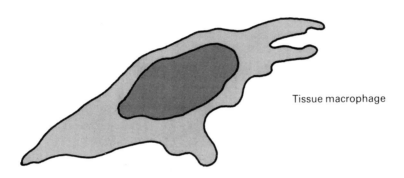

Tissue macrophage

The names given to macrophages in different tissues

Liver ———— Kupffer cell	Spleen ———— Dendritic cell
Connective tissue ———— Histiocyte	Nervous system ———— Microglial cell
Bone ———— Osteoclast	Lung ———— Alveolar macrophage

Cells mainly involved in non-specific immunity

Phagocytic cells

Mononuclear phagocytes

The mononuclear phagocytes include both circulating blood *monocytes* and *macrophages* found in various tissues of the body. The tissue macrophages are given special names depending on where they are.

The mononuclear phagocytes arise from bone marrow stem cells and, after proliferation and maturation, they pass into the blood as monocytes. After 24 hours they migrate to their main site of action in the tissues where they differentiate into macrophages. These are not end cells; they may divide, can synthesize protein, and are capable of surviving for many months.

Macrophages play a major role in *non-specific immunity* by their ability to ingest and destroy material such as bacteria, damaged host cells, or tumour cells.

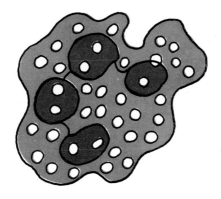

Polymorphonuclear
leucocyte
(neutrophil)
granules appear pale
pink on Leishman stain*

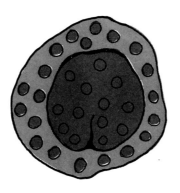

Eosinophil
leucocyte
granules appear red
on Leishman stain*

* The Leishman stain is commonly used in the microscopic
examination of blood films

Polymorphonuclear phagocytes (neutrophils)

Neutrophils are characterized by a large nucleus, usually with 3–5 lobes, and the presence of numerous granules in the cytoplasm.

Neutrophils arise from bone marrow stem cells common to mononuclear phagocytes, and approximately 50% of the mature cells are stored in the bone marrow ready to be called upon as needed to replenish cells in the circulation. After only about 12 hours in the blood, they enter the tissues where they complete their lifespan of a few days. They are *end cells* with no regenerative capacity.

The primary function of neutrophils is the *ingestion*, i.e. *phagocytosis*, and *killing* of invading micro-organisms, and the numbers of these cells in the peripheral blood generally increase markedly during the course of bacterial infections. They also play an important role in clearing the body of debris such as dead cells and thrombi.

Eosinophils

Eosinophils are easily distinguished by the presence of large granules in their cytoplasm which appear red when stained by routine staining techniques using *Leishman stain*. They are much less phagocytic than macrophages or neutrophils. The function of the eosinophil is far from clear; however, the numbers increase greatly in certain *parasitic diseases* such as worm infestation, and it is thought they have a role in defence against such infections. Their numbers are also increased during the course of certain types of *allergic disease*. Local tissue accumulations can occur in such conditions. For example, in asthma and hay fever large numbers of eosinophils may be found in the mucous membranes of the respiratory tract.

Both neutrophils and eosinophils contain *granules* in their cytoplasm. These granules contain various *enzymes* which are released under certain conditions.

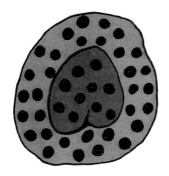

Basophil leucocyte
granules appear
dark bluish-purple
on Leishman stain

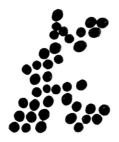

Platelets
dark bluish-purple
on Leishman stain

Mediator cells

The *mediator cells* influence the immune response by the release of various chemical substances into the circulation. These substances have a variety of biological activities including the ability to increase vascular permeability, contract smooth muscle, and enhance the inflammatory response. Basophils and platelets are found in the circulation, while mast cells are situated in the tissues of the skin, lung, and gastrointestinal tract.

Basophils and mast cells

Basophils are easily identified on a peripheral blood film by the appearance of large numbers of bluish-black granules in the cytoplasm. These granules are a source of mediators such as *histamine* and *heparin*. Circulating basophils greatly resemble tissue mast cells and it is likely that they are closely related in function.

Platelets

Platelets are small non-nucleated cells derived from *megakaryocytes* of the bone marrow. They are important in blood clotting. They probably also contribute to the immunological tissue injury occurring in certain types of hypersensitivity reactions by releasing *histamine* and related substances which are contained within specialized granules in their cytoplasm.

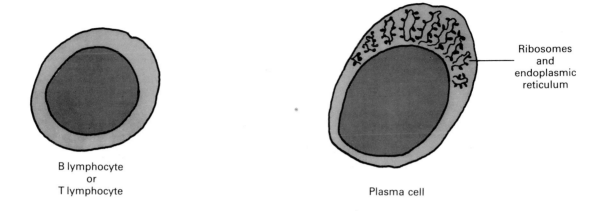

B lymphocyte
or
T lymphocyte

Ribosomes
and
endoplasmic
reticulum

Plasma cell

Normal numbers of cells in peripheral blood

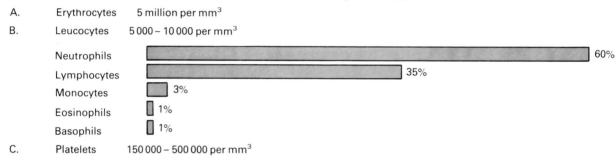

A.	Erythrocytes	5 million per mm^3
B.	Leucocytes	5 000 – 10 000 per mm^3
	Neutrophils	60%
	Lymphocytes	35%
	Monocytes	3%
	Eosinophils	1%
	Basophils	1%
C.	Platelets	150 000 – 500 000 per mm^3

Cells mainly involved in specific immunity

Cells of the *lymphoid cell line* differ from those previously described in that they have the ability to recognize certain substances (such as proteins) as *foreign* to the host and to eradicate them by means of the *specific immune response*. The host's own proteins, however, are not normally regarded as foreign and no specific response is mounted against them.

Lymphocytes

Traditionally, lymphocytes were classified morphologically into small, medium, and large. However, modern classification is based on function rather than appearance and every year more and more information is being obtained.

B lymphocytes are concerned with *humoral* immunity, i.e. they recognize certain substances as *foreign*, and when this recognition takes place the cells become metabolically very active, divide, and eventually become *plasma cells*. These in turn produce a family of proteins known as *antibodies* or *immunoglobulins*. B lymphocytes, plasma cells and their immunoglobulins are particularly important in the eradication of *circulating* foreign material such as bacteria.

B lymphocytes protect the host from bacterial infections.

T lymphocytes are not capable of differentiating into plasma cells and do not secrete antibody. However, they are important in recognizing foreign material that is *fixed in the tissues* or *inside cells*. Transplants, tumours, and the organisms causing tuberculosis are examples of such 'foreign' materials.

T lymphocytes protect the host from tumours and tuberculosis and are important in transplant rejection. (T lymphocytes are also important in *viral infections* but unfortunately this does not begin with a 'T'!)

(N.B. It is not possible to distinguish a T lymphocyte from a B lymphocyte from an ordinary blood film or tissue section. Special techniques are necessary.)

Plasma cells

Plasma cells have a large, eccentrically placed nucleus and a cytoplasm which is very rich in *ribonucleic acid* (RNA) and have an extensive system of *endoplasmic reticulum* and *ribosomes*. These structures are typical of cells engaged in very active protein synthesis—the protein in this instance being immunoglobulin.

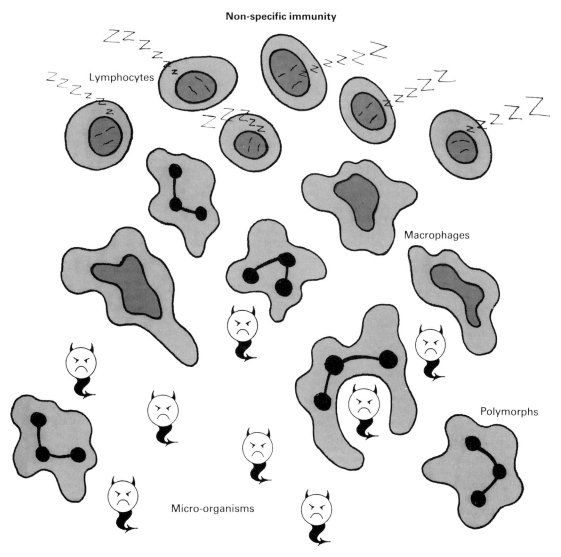

The cells mainly involved in an individual's **first** exposure to an antigen (e.g. microorganism) are polymorphs and macrophages. Lymphocytes are not fully involved until the **second** encounter (e.g. after immunization).

4. Non-specific immunity

Non-specific immunity is perhaps the most important body defence against infection. It is designed to give immediate protection on the *first* occasion the body meets any particular organism and it is active against a wide range of potentially infective agents. The cells involved in this first exposure are polymorphs and macrophages. Lymphocytes on the other hand come into play on *SECOND AND SUBSEQUENT* exposures and offer no real initial protection.

Certain factors may modify these defence mechanisms:

1. *Age*—Infectious diseases are more severe at the extremes of life. In babies this is partly associated with immaturity of the immune system, while in the elderly, underlying disorders (e.g. diabetes mellitus) and physical abnormalities (e.g. prostatic enlargement) lead to increased susceptibility to infection. In addition, the efficient functioning of

the immune system decreases with age.

2. *Hormones*—Certain hormones have been shown to affect the host's immune response. Steroids, for example, have an inhibitory effect on inflammation and antibody formation. Hypothyroidism and hypoadrenalism are associated with decreased resistance to infection.

3. *Drugs and chemicals*—Alcohol, for example, directly depresses the functioning of phagocytes. Some anaesthetic agents seem to have an inhibitory effect on phagocytes in the laboratory but it is not clear how important this is in a patient undergoing general anaesthesia.

4. *Malnutrition*—Poor nutrition is well known to be associated with increased susceptibility to infection.

The first line of defence—some physiological barriers

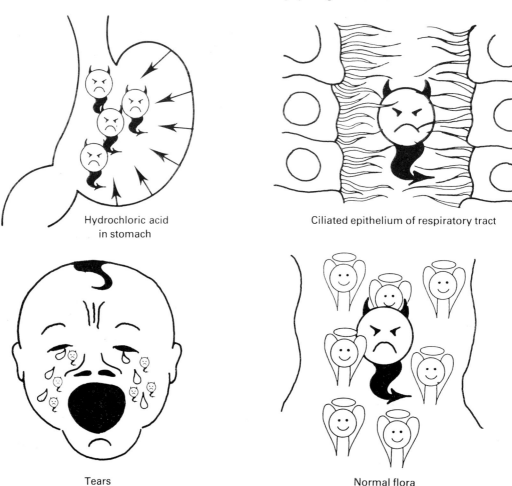

Hydrochloric acid
in stomach

Ciliated epithelium of respiratory tract

Tears

Normal flora

The first line of defence

The first line of defence that an invading microorganism meets is the *physical barrier* provided by the intact skin and mucous membranes. The skin is the more resistant because of its outer horny layer. However, when the integrity of the skin is broken by, for example, burns, eczema, or surgical incision, invasion by microorganisms may result.

The body enhances its defence against bacterial invasion by certain *physiological factors*. For example:

1. *Hydrochloric acid* in the stomach destroys many ingested organisms. This protective mechanism is absent in patients with pernicious anaemia who have achlorhydria.

2. The *ciliated epithelium* lining the respiratory tract traps and sweeps away inhaled bacteria. Smokers often have damaged respiratory epithelium and so this mechanism is less efficient than in the non-smoker.
3. The *flushing action of urine* helps prevent the establishment of infection in the urinary tract. Urinary tract infection is well known to be associated with urinary stasis, e.g. in ureteric reflux, bladder tumour, neurological abnormalities leading to sphincter disturbance.
4. The large amounts of *unsaturated fatty acids* found in the *skin* are known to kill bacteria, while *sweat* contains appreciable quantities of *salt* which is inhibitory to many bacteria which would otherwise reside in the skin.

5. *Human tears* contain large quantities of *lysozyme*, an enzyme which can destroy bacteria. Lysozyme is also found in other body fluids, e.g. saliva, intestinal mucus, nasal secretions, and is present in high concentrations in neutrophils.
6. The *normal commensal flora* is in itself an important defence mechanism. Skin, for example, is normally colonized with relatively harmless organisms such as *Staphylococcus albus* and diphtheroids. The mouth and throat are inhabited mainly by *Streptococcus viridans*, and the colon contains a whole host of organisms such as bacteroides, coliforms, streptococci, and clostridial species. This well-balanced mixture of organisms can exert a protective effect by preventing excessive overgrowth by potentially more harmful organisms.

Normal inflammatory response

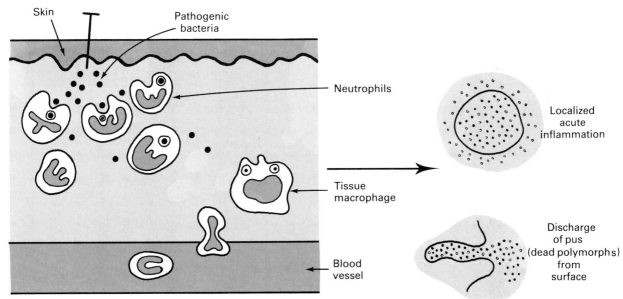

The second line of defence

If the invading organism gets through the first line of defence and enters the tissues, further non-specific host responses are stimulated, i.e. the *inflammatory response* and *phagocytosis*. The organisms may be engulfed by wandering tissue macrophages or they may trigger the inflammatory response bringing neutrophils from the blood to the site of infection. The inflammatory response consists of local dilation of capillaries, slowing of the blood flow, and the exudation of phagocytic cells and serum bactericidal factors. Once outside the capillaries the neutrophils migrate to the source of infection. This phenomenon is known as *chemotaxis*, i.e. *unidirectional locomotion towards an increasing gradient of attractant*, which in this situation is the breakdown products of damaged tissue cells. The neutrophils then attach

to and ingest the organisms (phagocytosis). Once ingested, susceptible bacteria are killed by acids and digestive enzymes secreted by the neutrophils.

If bacteria are not successfully killed locally, they may further invade the host by way of the lymphatics to the *regional lymph nodes*. Within the lymph nodes the bacteria meet other phagocytic cells (*macrophages*).

Bacteria may overcome these local and lymphatic-associated barriers and gain access to the *blood stream*. Here they meet *circulating* phagocytes (*neutrophils and monocytes*), or they may reach organs such as the *liver* and *spleen* where they come into contact with *tissue macrophages*.

Although a powerful defence system, this final phagocytic barrier may be overcome, with seeding of the microorganisms to organs such as bone, brain, and kidney, terminating in fatal septicaemia.

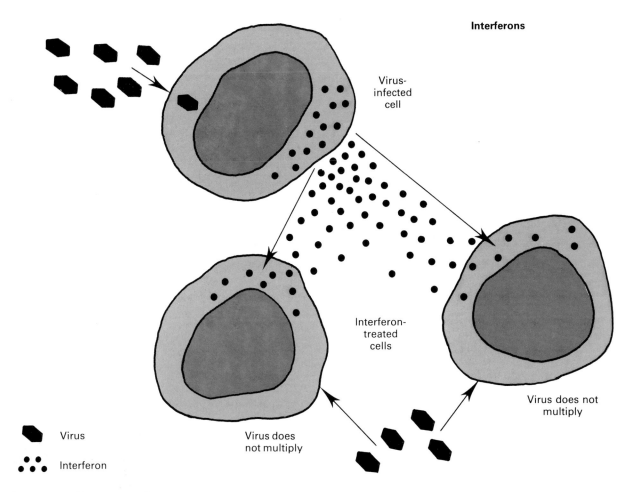

Interferons

Virus-
infected
cell

Interferon-
treated
cells

Virus does not
multiply

Virus does
not multiply

Virus

Interferon

Serum factors that are damaging to microorganisms

Many soluble tissue and serum substances help to suppress the growth of, or kill, microorganisms. The following are some examples:

1. *Interferons*—These are a family of proteins which are important in the non-specific defence mechanisms against *viral infection*. They are released from virus-infected cells and, when taken up by other cells, protect them from infection not only from the virus in question, but also from other types of virus. They are probably the main factor responsible for recovery from acute viral infection. In recent years it has been shown that macrophages and T lymphocytes also produce interferon, and much research is being carried out in this area. In view of the fact that antibiotics are ineffective in the treatment of viral disease, it was hoped that interferon could be used as a therapeutic agent. This has not yet been shown to be the case. There is, however, evidence that it may prove to be helpful in the management of some types of tumour.

2. *Transferrin*—Bacteria are dependent on iron for their multiplication and they have to compete with iron-binding proteins in the patient's serum. Such a protein is *transferrin*. Bacteria do not thrive well in serum that contains low levels of iron but high levels of transferrin. In such serum the iron is not available for bacterial growth. Conversely, low transferrin levels probably contribute to the susceptibility to infection seen in malnutrition, since the patient's iron is accessible to the micro-organism.

3. *Complement*—A group of proteins that we know as *complement* is essential for bacterial destruction and plays an important role in both non-specific and specific immune mechanisms. Complement will be discussed later.

The body's first encounter with a pathogenic organism stimulates, therefore, the non-specific defence system but, as we shall see later, there is participation also by the '*third line of defence*'—the *specific immune system*. This is important in protection against infection when the host is subsequently exposed to the microorganism.

Phagocytosis

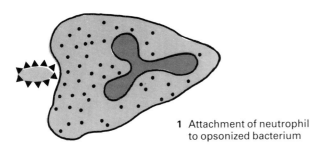

1 Attachment of neutrophil to opsonized bacterium

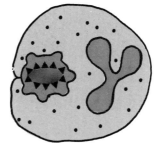

3 Discharge of granule contents into vacuole (degranulation)

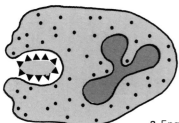

2 Engulfment of bacterium

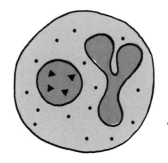

4 Killing and digestion of bacterium inside phagocytic vacuole

Phagocytosis

The phagocytosis and killing of bacteria is an extremely important defence mechanism of the body against infection and is therefore worthy of further attention.

As previously mentioned, phagocytic cells are of two types, the neutrophils in the blood and the monocytes and macrophages distributed throughout the body both circulating in the blood and fixed in the tissues.

Phagocytosis, the process by which a particle is ingested by a cell, can be divided into two stages:

1. The *attachment phase*.
2. The *ingestion phase*.

During the *attachment phase*, firm contact is made between the phagocyte and microorganism. As we shall see later, this is enhanced when the antigen is coated by its specific antibody and complement, i.e. it is *opsonized*.

The *ingestion phase* represents engulfment of the organism, which is taken up into the cytoplasm of the phagocyte and enclosed within a pocket (*vacuole*). Some of the cytoplasmic granules within the phagocyte come into close contact with this vacuole. The granules rupture, discharging their damaging enzymatic contents into the vacuole and so destroying the microorganism.

There are a number of killing mechanisms operating in the vacuoles of phagocytic cells. One of the major mechanisms involves *hydrogen peroxide* which, acting alone with an intracellular enzyme, is rapidly lethal to many bacteria.

Natural killer cells

Natural killer (NK) cells look like lymphocytes but are of uncertain origin. They are *cytotoxic cells*, i.e. they have the capacity to bind to and destroy certain other target cells, particularly *tumour* and *virus-infected cells*. NK cells are activated by interferons (which, as mentioned previously, are themselves components of the non-specific immune system).

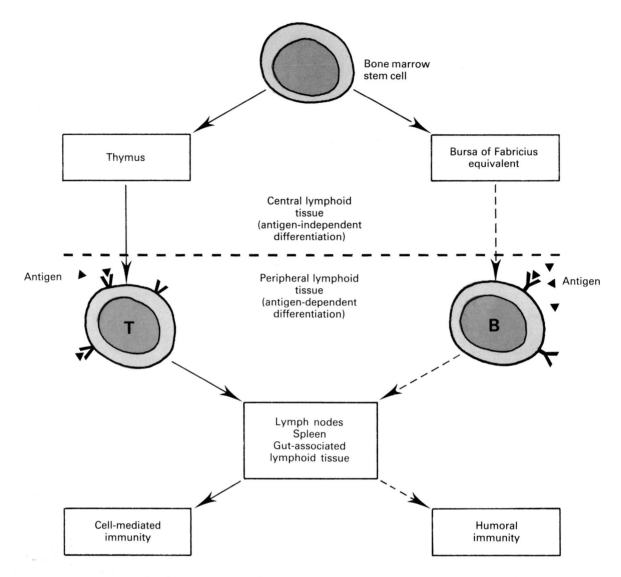

5. Organs of the specific immune system
Specific immunity

Non-specific immune mechanisms deal with potentially harmful materials on the host's *first* and *subsequent exposures* to them. On the other hand, *specific immune responses*, although they may play a part in the recovery phase after infection has taken place, *offer no immediate protection on the first occasion a host meets a particular antigen, but they are effective on second and subsequent exposures*. This phenomenon is illustrated during the course of natural infections or immunization. Measles, for example, is a viral infection which generally results in clinical infection during childhood after first exposure to the virus. The host's non-specific defence mechanisms are generally not effective in preventing infection. However, on second and subsequent exposures the specific immune system is brought rapidly into play. This offers a high degree of protection and as a result second attacks of measles are extremely rare.

Specific immunity results from activity of cells and organs of the *lymphoid system*, whch consists of two components:

1. A *central component* involved in the differentiation of stem cells into lymphocytes capable of reacting with antigen. This differentiation can occur in the absence of antigen.

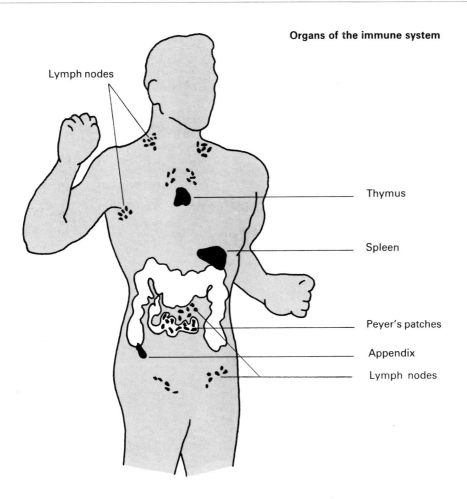

Organs of the immune system

Lymph nodes

Thymus

Spleen

Peyer's patches

Appendix

Lymph nodes

2. A *peripheral component* in which these cells react with antigen and differentiate further. This step is antigen-dependent.

The *central lymphoid system* consists of:

A. *Bone marrow.*
B. *Thymus.*
C. A component whose identity is known with certainty only in birds—*the bursa of Fabricius*. In mammals it is known as *bursal equivalent tissue* but its site is not clear.

The *peripheral lymphoid system* consists of:

A. *Lymph nodes.*
B. *Spleen.*

C. The *gut-associated lymphoid tissue*, namely Peyer's patches and the appendix.

Two types of lymphocytes (T and B) are found in the peripheral lymphoid tissues. They are named according to their site of differentiation in the central lymphoid compartment.

1. $\boxed{T}$ *lymphocytes* develop in the $\boxed{t}$*hymus* and are involved in antigen recognition in *cell-mediated immune reactions.*
2. $\boxed{B}$ *lymphocytes* differentiate in the $\boxed{b}$*ursal equivalent tissue* and are involved in the production of antibody, i.e. *humoral immunity.*

Organization of the thymus

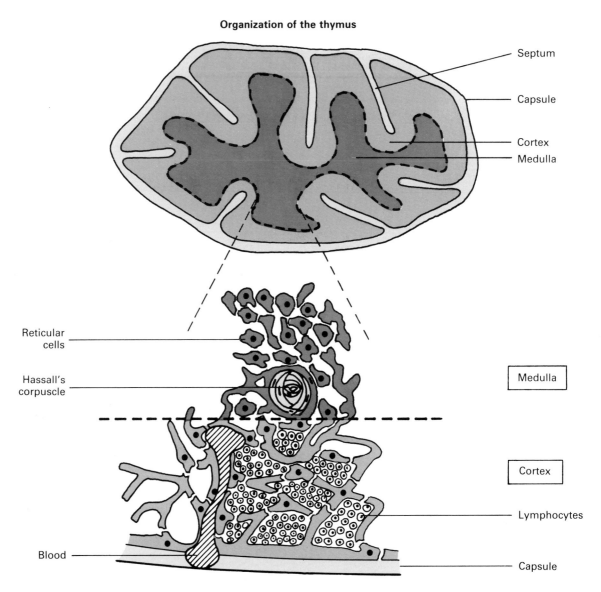

(*Hassall's corpuscles* are a feature peculiar to the medulla of the thymus and consist of groups of reticular cells sometimes flattened and concentrically arranged around a central core of nuclear debris. Reticular cells make up the framework of lymphoid tissues throughout the body)

Organs of the immune system

The main organs of the immune system are the *thymus, spleen* and *lymph nodes.* In addition, there is *lymphoid tissue* scattered throughout the gastrointestinal, respiratory, and urinary tracts.

Thymus

The thymus, in man, is the central lymphoid organ upon which other peripheral organs are dependent.

Relative to body size, it is largest during foetal life and in the young child. The organ continues to increase in size until puberty. Following adolescence, it slowly atrophies although it is still readily visible in the adult.

The thymus consists of two lobes surrounded by a capsule. The outer part is heavily infiltrated with *thymocytes*, morphologically similar to blood lymphocytes.

The main function of the thymus is to stimulate differentiation and proliferation of primitive bone marrow derived lymphoid cells. It is likely that this is achieved via production of a hormone.

Experimentally, if the thymus is removed during the neonatal period, certain areas of the lymph nodes and spleen become deficient in lymphocytes and the animals have impaired cell-mediated immune responses.

Organization of a lymph node

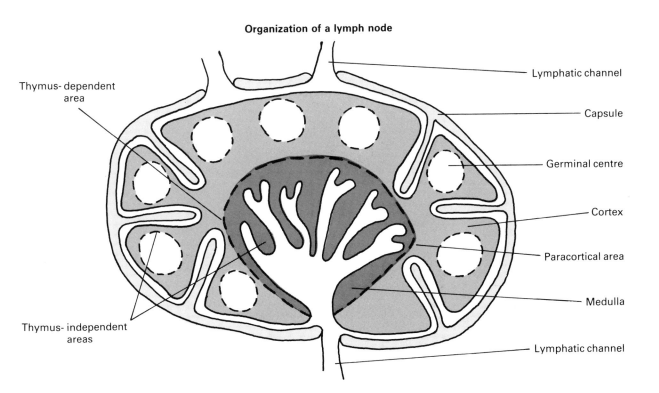

Thymus-dependent area

Lymphatic channel

Capsule

Germinal centre

Cortex

Paracortical area

Medulla

Thymus-independent areas

Lymphatic channel

Lymph nodes and spleen

These are capsulated organs of the peripheral lymphoid system through which foreign materials in the lymph and blood must pass and come into contact with macrophages and lymphocytes. They are important centres for phagocytosis and for the initiation and development of specific responses of humoral and cell-mediated immunity. Their structure, therefore, can be thought of as a complex organization of the three types of cell chiefly involved in these processes, i.e. macrophages, lymphocytes, and plasma cells.

Lymph nodes

Lymph is a collection of tissue fluid flowing from the limbs and tissues through the lymph nodes on its way to the blood stream via the largest lymph channel—the *thoracic duct*. The tissue of a lymph node is organized into an outer *cortex* and an inner *medulla*. The cortex is made up of large numbers of lymphocytes organized into areas known as *nodules*. In the centre of these nodules collections of actively dividing cells of the B lymphocyte line develop in response to antigenic stimulation. These areas are known as *germinal centres*. Other regions of the lymph node known as the *paracortical areas* are populated with T lymphocytes which are under the control of the thymus.

Organization of the spleen

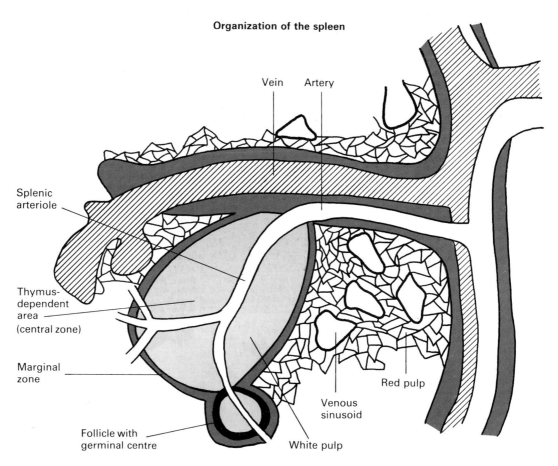

Vein   Artery

Splenic
arteriole

Thymus-
dependent
area
(central zone)

Marginal
zone

Follicle with
germinal centre

White pulp

Venous
sinusoid

Red pulp

Spleen

The spleen is the only lymphatic tissue specialized to filter blood. The tissues of the interior are organized into *white pulp* and *red pulp*. As in the lymph node, the T and B areas are segregated. The *central zone* contains T lymphocytes—the thymus-dependent area. The *marginal zone* contains B lymphocytes and plasma cells.

The *red pulp* consists of blood vessels lined with macrophages.

Main immunological functions of the lymph nodes and spleen

1. *The removal of particulate matter from blood and lymph.* Foreign material is filtered from the lymph as it passes through the lymph nodes, and from the blood as it passes through the red pulp of the spleen. The foreign material comes into contact with large numbers of phagocytic cells and may be removed from the circulation.
2. *Specific response to circulating antigens.* Both lymph nodes and spleen are capable of responding to circulating antigens with the production of specific lymphocytes and plasma cells leading to the initiation of the specific immune response.

Unencapsulated lymphoid tissue

The respiratory, alimentary and genitourinary tracts are 'guarded' immunologically by subepithelial accumulations of lymphoid tissue. These may occur as diffuse collections of lymphocytes, plasma cells, and phagocytes or as more clearly organized tissue known as *follicles*, e.g. the tonsils, Peyer's patches, and appendix.

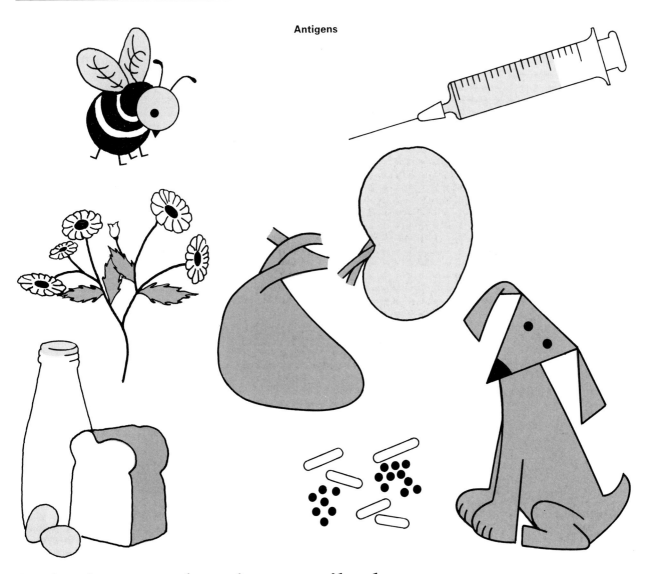

6. Antigens and antigen–antibody binding

Antigens

An *antigen* is any substance which is capable, under appropriate conditions, of provoking a specific immune response. It is capable of:

A. Stimulating the formation of antibody and the development of cell-mediated immunity.

B. Reacting *specifically* with the antibodies or T lymphocytes produced.

(N.B. 'Specific' means here that the antigen will react in a highly selective fashion with the corresponding antibody and not with a multitude of other antibodies evoked by other antigens.)

A *hapten* is a substance, usually of low molecular weight, that can combine with antibody but cannot initiate an immune response unless it is coupled to a larger *carrier* molecule. For example, nickel is a substance of small molecular weight which is incapable of provoking an immune response in its own right. Nickel allergy, however, is a common cause of contact dermatitis. This results when nickel combines with protein in the patient's skin. The nickel–protein complex is recognized as foreign and an immune response is mounted.

Generally, the most potent antigens are *proteins* or *polysaccharides*. Not all the factors that make a substance antigenic have been identified, but certain basic properties are known to be essential.

Factors influencing antigenicity

An important prerequisite for antigenicity is that the substance is *foreign* to the body. The immune system of an individual can normally distinguish between body components, i.e. '*self*', and foreign substances, '*non-self*'. Normally, the body is *tolerant* to its own components and does not initiate an immune response against these. Under certain circumstances, however, this natural tolerance may be disturbed, permitting the individual to react against himself, as is seen in *autoimmune disease*.

Molecular size is an important factor. Small molecules such as amino acids or monosaccharides are usually not antigenic. As a rule, molecules with a molecular weight of less than 10,000 have no or only weak antigenicity. However, as mentioned above, if coupled to a suitable carrier molecule such as a protein, low molecular weight substances (haptens) can exhibit antigenicity.

The *configuration* and *complexity* of the molecule are important. Linear polypeptides and globular proteins are both capable of inducing an immune response. Antibody that is formed to these different structures is highly specific and when the conformation of an antigen is changed the antibody induced by the original form no longer combines with it. For example, it is possible for an individual to produce an immune response to raw egg antigens, but when the egg is boiled the antigenic configuration is changed and no immune response is mounted. The need for complexity means that molecules containing a repeating unit of only one amino acid are generally poor antigens, even if the molecule is large.

Genetic factors also play a part. Not all individuals within a species will show the same response to a substance—some are *responders* and some *nonresponders*. Likewise, there is a wide variation between species.

The *method of administration* and the *dose* are also important. The immune response to a substance can be enhanced by administering an *adjuvant** together with the antigen, while a state of *immunological unresponsiveness* can result if very high or very low doses of certain antigens are administered.

Factors influencing antigenicity

- Foreign nature
- Molecular size
- Molecular complexity and rigidity
- Genetic factors in the individual
- Method of administration
- Dosage

---

* An *adjuvant* is a substance injected with antigens which non-specifically enhances the immune response to that antigen.

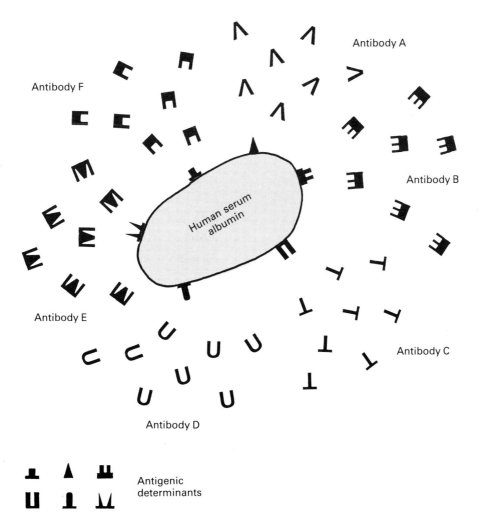

Diversity of antibody induced by one antigen

Antibody A

Antibody F

Antibody B

Human serum albumin

Antibody E

Antibody C

Antibody D

Antigenic determinants

Antigenic determinants

Despite the fact that potent antigens are relatively large molecules, only limited parts of the molecule are involved in the binding to antibodies. These parts are called *antigenic determinants* or *epitopes*. A molecule must have at least two antigenic determinants in order to stimulate antibody production.

The number of antigenic determinants on a molecule varies with molecular size. Human albumin, for example, has at least six different antigenic determinants, which means that at least six antibodies of different specificities can be produced after immunization of, for example, a rabbit.

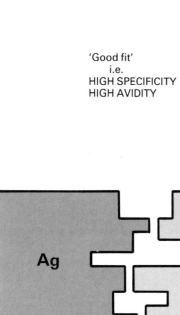

'Good fit'
i.e.
HIGH SPECIFICITY
HIGH AVIDITY

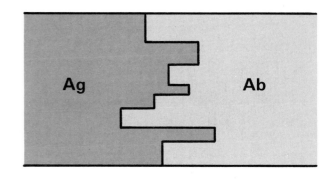

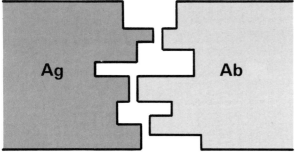

No reaction between
antigen and antibody
i.e. the ANTIBODY
COMBINING SITE does not
fit the ANTIGENIC
DETERMINANT

'Poor fit'
i.e.
LOWER SPECIFICITY
LOW AVIDITY

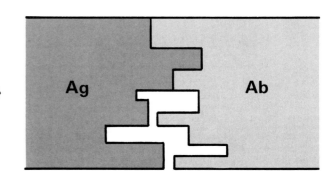

Antigen–antibody binding

The binding of the *antigenic determinant* to the *antibody binding site* can be likened to a 'lock and key' situation. The most efficient immunological responses occur when the antigen and antibody fit exactly. Antibodies of different degrees of specificity may be produced in the immune response to a given antigen.

Sometimes an antigen can combine as a 'poor fit' with an antibody that was produced in response to an entirely different antigen. This is demonstrated in the phenomenon of *cross-reactivity*. In the course of some infections, antibody produced to the microorganism in question can produce a 'poor fit' with the host's own tissue antigens and immunological damage may result. For example, in acute rheumatic fever, it is thought that antibody produced against *Streptococcus pyogenes* in the throat cross-reacts with the host's heart tissue leading to myocarditis and valvular disease.

Basic four-chain structure

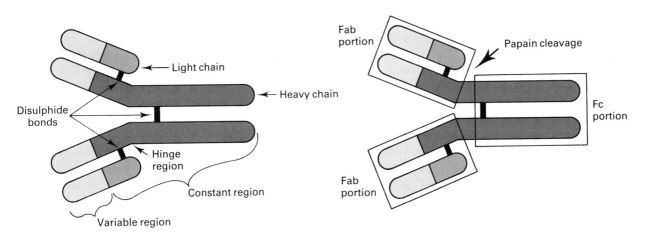

7. Immunoglobulins

Basic structure

The basic immunoglobulin unit consists of two identical *heavy chains* and two *light chains*, held together by a chemical link (disulphide bonds). Light chains are named by the greek letters *kappa* (κ) and *lambda* (λ), and the heavy chains by *gamma* (γ), *alpha* (α), *mu* (μ), *delta* (δ), and *epsilon* (ε). The various immunoglobulin classes are distinguished by their heavy chains. Only one type of light chain is found in any individual molecule.

Papain, a protein-digesting enzyme, splits the antibody molecule into three large pieces. Two of the pieces are identical and contain the *antibody binding site*. These have been termed the antibody binding fragment or *Fab fragment*. They are composed of the entire light chain and about half of the heavy chain linked to each other by a disulphide bond. The Fab portions contain what is known as the '*variable*' regions of the molecule in which the amino acid sequence is very different from molecule to molecule. It is this variable region that provides the 'lock' of the antibody molecule, i.e. it is highly specific for the binding of one particular antibody to an antigen. The third fragment plays no part in combining with antigen but has many other important functions; for example, the structure of this site determines whether the antibody will cross the placenta or take part in complement fixation (see later). When the molecule is chemically split, this fragment can be obtained in a crystalline form; therefore, it is termed the *Fc fragment*.

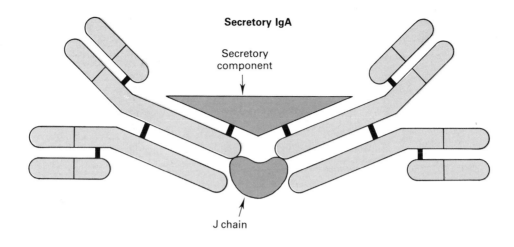

Secretory IgA

Secretory
component

J chain

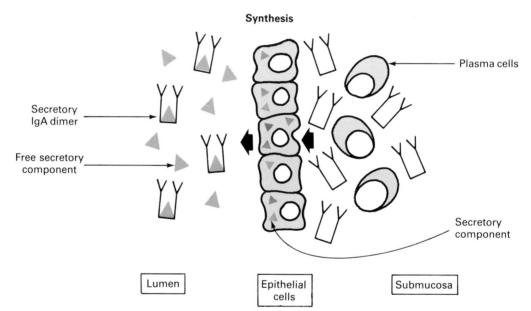

Synthesis

Plasma cells

Secretory
IgA dimer

Free secretory
component

Secretory
component

Lumen | Epithelial cells | Submucosa

Classification of immunoglobulins

In man five different classes of immunoglobulin are known to exist, each with a distinct chemical structure and a specific biological role.

IgG

This is the most abundant of the immunoglobulins in the plasma and because of its relatively small molecular weight it can diffuse into the interstitial fluid. It is therefore found in significant concentrations in both vascular and extravascular spaces and plays a major role in the defence against both blood-borne infective agents and those invading the tissues.

The complexes of microorganism with IgG antibody activate the complement system and thereby attract polymorphs to the site of infection. IgG can also coat organisms and this enhances their phagocytosis by neutrophils and macrophages.

Through its ability to cross the placenta, maternal IgG provides the major line of defence against infection for the first few weeks of a baby's life.

IgA

As well as being present in the serum, IgA is the major immunoglobulin of the external secretory system and is found in saliva, tears, colostrum, and breast milk, and in nasal, bronchial and intestinal secretions. It is produced in high concentrations by lymphoid tissues lining the gastrointestinal, respira-

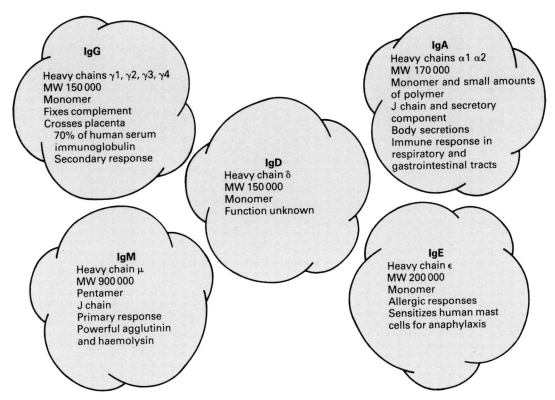

IgG
Heavy chains γ1, γ2, γ3, γ4
MW 150 000
Monomer
Fixes complement
Crosses placenta
70% of human serum
immunoglobulin
Secondary response

IgD
Heavy chain δ
MW 150 000
Monomer
Function unknown

IgA
Heavy chains α1 α2
MW 170 000
Monomer and small amounts
of polymer
J chain and secretory
component
Body secretions
Immune response in
respiratory and
gastrointestinal tracts

IgM
Heavy chain μ
MW 900 000
Pentamer
J chain
Primary response
Powerful agglutinin
and haemolysin

IgE
Heavy chain ε
MW 200 000
Monomer
Allergic responses
Sensitizes human mast
cells for anaphylaxis

tory, and genitourinary tracts, and it is likely that it plays an important role in protection against respiratory, urinary tract and bowel infections. It is probably also important in preventing absorption of potential antigens in the food we eat.

In serum, IgA exists as a single molecule or as two or three molecules joined together. The IgA present in secretions, however, exists as two molecules (a *dimer*) attached to another molecule known as *secretory component*. This substance is produced by the cells lining the mucous membranes and is thought to protect the IgA in secretions from destruction by digestive enzymes.

IgA does not cross the placenta. However, it is present in large quantities in colostrum and breast milk. Thus, it probably plays an important role in protecting the neonate from infection—hence the importance of breast feeding. Serum IgA is the last immunoglobulin to develop in childhood, although secretory IgA tends to appear early.

IgM

This is a large molecule consisting of five of the basic units (a *pentamer*) joined together by a structure known as *J-chain*. IgM is restricted almost entirely to the intravascular space due to its large size.

IgM is the first antibody to be produced and is of greatest importance early in the immune response

to an infecting organism. It acts as an effective means of defence during the bacteraemic phase of an infection.

IgD

This immunoglobulin normally occurs in small amounts in the serum. It has been found on the surface of lymphocytes, but little is known about the function of this class of antibody.

IgE

The concentration of IgE in the serum is normally very low, only about 0.004% of the total immunoglobulins. Elevated levels of IgE are normally found in patients suffering from *atopic* disease such as asthma and hay fever (see p. 48). Certain cells, i.e. mast cells and basophils, possess receptors for the Fc fragment of IgE, and as a consequence, a certain amount of IgE is bound to these cells. On contact with a specific antigen, the cell-bound IgE antibodies mediate the release of pharmacologically active substances from the cells, resulting in the allergic symptoms. The normal biological role of IgE is still uncertain, however. It is thought that IgE may be important in the defence against *parasitic infections* since elevated IgE levels are noted in such cases.

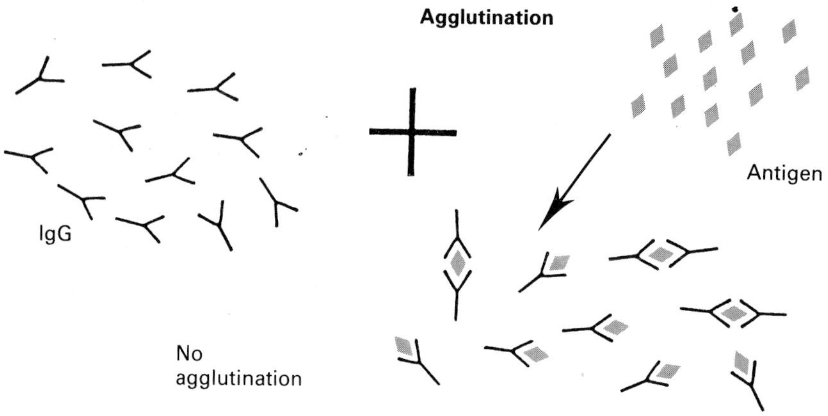

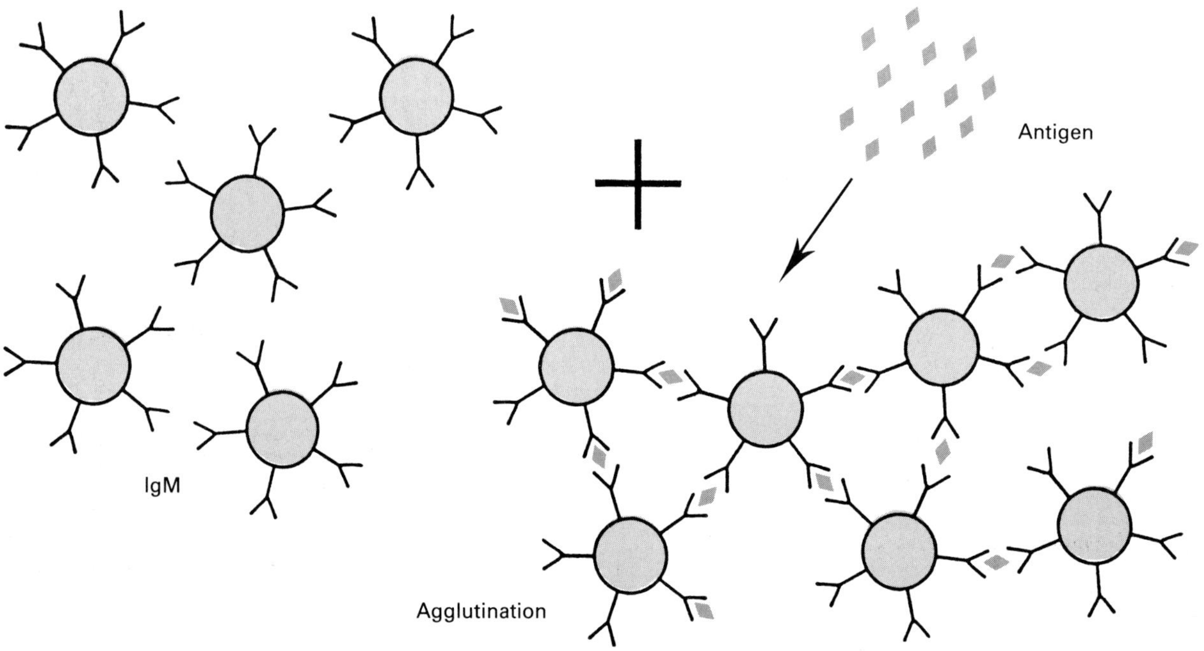

Agglutination

IgG

No agglutination

Antigen

IgM

Antigen

Agglutination

Agglutination

As already mentioned, antibody molecules have at least two combining sites—the Fab portions. The antibody, therefore, can act as a cross-link between two antigens, e.g. red blood cells or bacteria, and bind them or clump them together. This clumping is called *agglutination*.

IgM is the most powerful agglutinating class of antibody; it is about one thousand times as efficient as

IgG. This is because of the many combining sites present in one IgM pentamer. The prime function, therefore, of the IgM class of antibody is the agglutination and clearing of any bacteria invading the blood stream.

(Agglutination is also the basis for many useful laboratory tests such as blood grouping.)

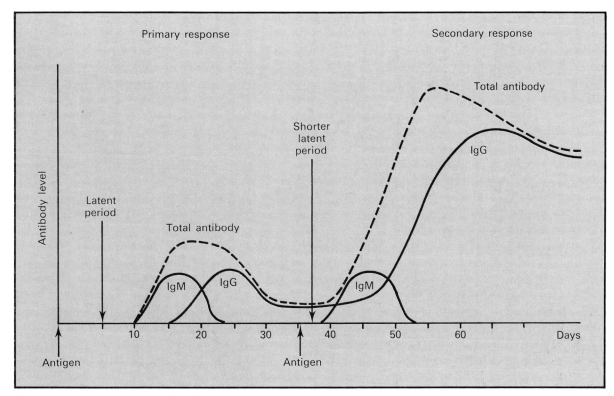

The primary and secondary antibody responses

8. The humoral immune response

The dynamics of antibody production

(i) Total antibody levels

Exposure to antigen is followed by a latent period during which there is no detectable antibody. On first exposure to antigen the latent period of several days is followed by the *primary response*. There is a rapid rise in serum antibody for a few days only and then the specific antibody concentrations reach a plateau and over the succeeding weeks diminish to very low or undetectable levels.

After the primary response there is a prolonged phase of *immunological memory* DURING WHICH THERE IS ENHANCED SECONDARY RESPONSE TO THE ADMINISTRATION OF ANTIGEN. This memory lasts for many years and may be lifelong.

The secondary response is characterized by a shorter latent period, faster production and higher concentration of antibody.

(ii) IgM and IgG components of the humoral immune response

There are qualitative differences in the antibody produced at various times during the immune response. In the primary response, the initial antibody is IgM and its production lasts 10–12 days. Thereafter in the absence of continued antigenic stimulus, IgM antibody disappears. An IgG response follows with large quantities of IgG being produced for several months.

In the secondary response, specific IgM is produced but the bulk of the increased antibody production is IgG.

In natural infections, because the organisms are multiplying a large mass of antigen builds up and acts as a stimulus over a number of days. In this situation the classical primary and secondary immune responses are indistinguishable and both occur on initial exposure to antigen.

Because specific IgM, unlike IgG, does *not* remain elevated long after the antigenic stimulus has been removed, it is an important indicator of *present* or *very recent* INFECTION.

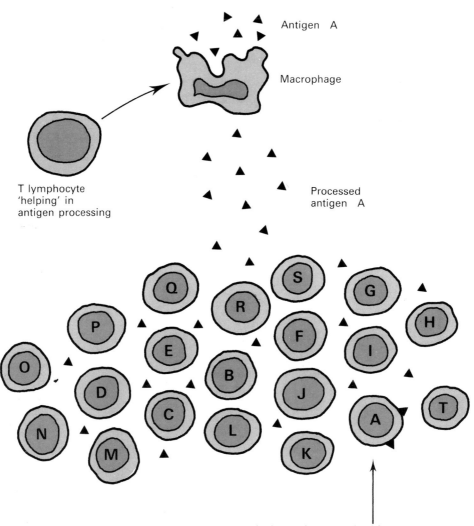

Stimulation of specific B cells

Antigen A

Macrophage

T lymphocyte 'helping' in antigen processing

Processed antigen A

Antigen A recognized by an 'appropriate' B lymphocyte. Other lymphocytes 'ignore' this antigen

Cellular events in antibody production

(i) Stimulation of specific B cells

Antigen is first 'processed' by macrophages so that it can be presented in a suitable form to the circulating pool of B lymphocytes. Sometimes, the *help* of a special type of T lymphocyte is required in the processing of certain antigens. This emphasizes the need for *cooperation* between the various sections of the immune system.

A small number of cells in the B lymphocyte pool have *specific receptors* for the antigen in question. Reaction between receptor and antigen stimulates B cell division in that group of cells only. All other B cells 'programmed' to recognize different antigens will *not* be 'stimulated' to divide.

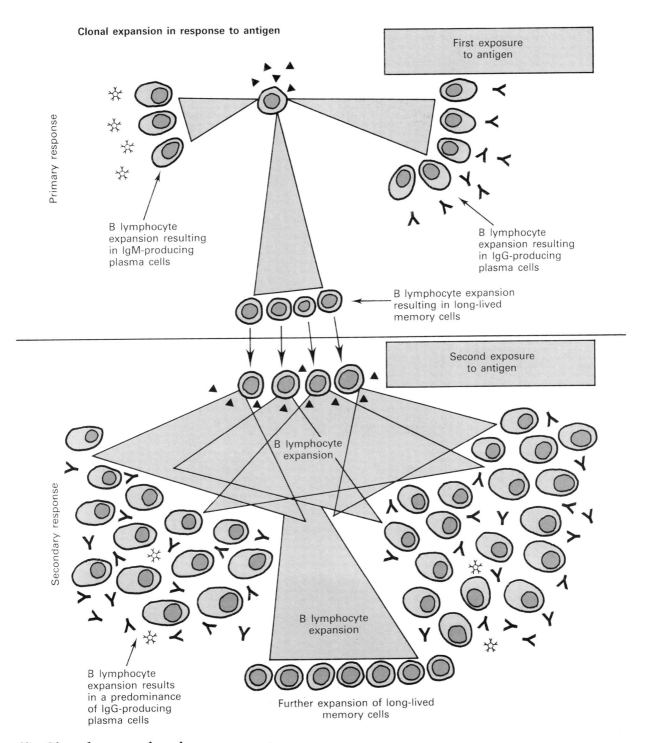

Clonal expansion in response to antigen

First exposure to antigen

Primary response

B lymphocyte expansion resulting in IgM-producing plasma cells

B lymphocyte expansion resulting in IgG-producing plasma cells

B lymphocyte expansion resulting in long-lived memory cells

Second exposure to antigen

B lymphocyte expansion

Secondary response

B lymphocyte expansion

B lymphocyte expansion results in a predominance of IgG-producing plasma cells

Further expansion of long-lived memory cells

(ii) Clonal expansion in response to antigen

The result of B lymphocyte cell division triggered by antigenic exposure is the production of a *clone* of B cells, all with identical characteristics and antigenic specificity. Some of these lymphocytes become plasma cells capable of producing IgM. Later IgG-producing plasma cells appear.

In addition to B lymphocytes destined to become plasma cells, another group of lymphocytes known as *memory cells* appear. When the antigenic stimulus is removed, cell division and differentiation stop but the circulating pool of lymphocytes now contain a large population of memory cells to that particular antigen. These are extremely long-lived (many years) and when the same antigen is encountered on second and subsequent occasions they are responsible for more rapid and extensive cell division and differentiation into IgG-producing plasma cells, i.e. the SECONDARY RESPONSE.

(iii) Heavy chain switching

During the course of maturation from stem cell to plasma cell, B lymphocytes undergo several changes. One of these changes involves the appearance and disappearance of different classes of immunoglobulin bound to their surface membranes. These membrane-bound immunoglobulins are slightly different chemically from those eventually secreted by plasma cells.

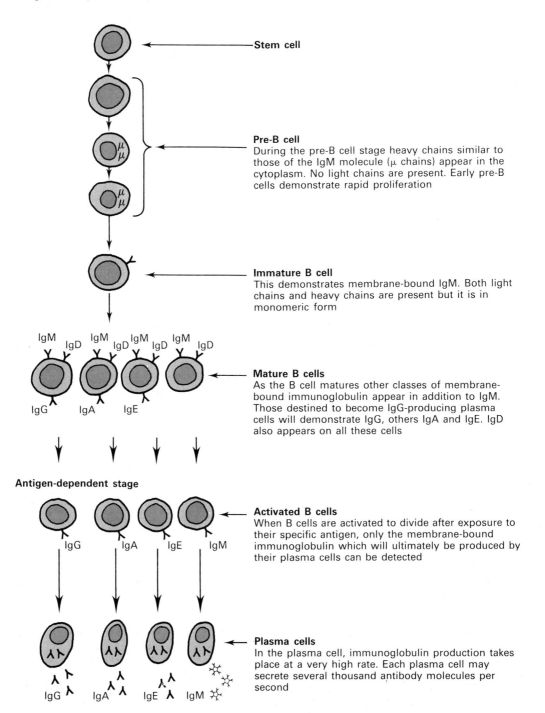

Antigen – independent stage

Stem cell

Pre-B cell
During the pre-B cell stage heavy chains similar to those of the IgM molecule (μ chains) appear in the cytoplasm. No light chains are present. Early pre-B cells demonstrate rapid proliferation

Immature B cell
This demonstrates membrane-bound IgM. Both light chains and heavy chains are present but it is in monomeric form

IgM IgD IgM IgD IgM IgD IgM IgD
IgG IgA IgE

Mature B cells
As the B cell matures other classes of membrane-bound immunoglobulin appear in addition to IgM. Those destined to become IgG-producing plasma cells will demonstrate IgG, others IgA and IgE. IgD also appears on all these cells

Antigen-dependent stage

IgG IgA IgE IgM

Activated B cells
When B cells are activated to divide after exposure to their specific antigen, only the membrane-bound immunoglobulin which will ultimately be produced by their plasma cells can be detected

IgG IgA IgE IgM

Plasma cells
In the plasma cell, immunoglobulin production takes place at a very high rate. Each plasma cell may secrete several thousand antibody molecules per second

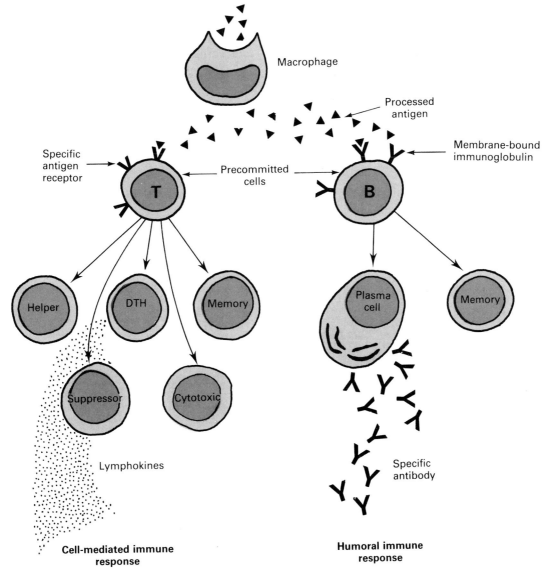

Cell-mediated immune response

Humoral immune response

9. The cellular immune response

Cell-mediated immunity

Cell-mediated immunity is important in defence against viral infections, some fungal infections, parasitic disease and against some bacteria, particularly those inside cells. In these situations the antigen is physically and architecturally inaccessible and antigen–antibody reactions appear to be relatively inefficient.

Cell-mediated immunity is also responsible for delayed hypersensitivity, transplant rejection and, probably, is involved in tumour surveillance.

The integrity of this branch of the immune system depends on the presence of thymus-derived lymphocytes (T lymphocytes).

A cell-mediated reaction is initiated by the binding of antigen with an antigen receptor on the surface of a sensitized T lymphocyte. The nature of the T cell receptor is still being investigated. Unlike the B cell receptor, this is *not* an immunoglobulin molecule but nonetheless it incorporates a structure similar to the Fab region of the immunoglobulin. This antigen T cell binding may occur directly or be mediated by macrophages. The reaction stimulates differentiation of the T lymphocytes into two main groups of cells:

1. *Helper* and *suppressor T cells* that regulate the height of the body's immune responses.
2. T cells capable of *direct interaction* with the antigen.

The latter group is further divisible into:

A. T cells which, on contact with specific antigen, are responsible for delayed type hypersensitivity by liberating substances called *lymphokines*.
B. *Cytotoxic T cells* which directly attack antigen on the surface of foreign cells.

Lymphokines are a mixed group of proteins. Very few have been identified chemically, and most can only be classified in terms of their biological activities. They have diverse properties, but *macrophages* are probably the principal target cells. Some lymphokines will aggregate macrophages at the site of the infection, while others activate macrophages, inducing them to phagocytose and destroy foreign antigens more vigorously. A further important function is the attraction of neutrophils and monocytes to the site of infection. In short, the end result of their combined action is an amplification of the local inflammatory reaction with recruitment of circulating cells of the immune system.

Contact between antigen and *specific* sensitized T cells is necessary to cause release of lymphokines, but once released the lymphokine action is *not antigen-specific*; for example, an immune reaction to the tubercle bacillus may protect an animal against simultaneous challenge by brucella organisms.

Cytotoxic T cells, on the other hand, attach directly to the target cell via specific receptors. The target cell is lysed; the cytotoxic cell is not destroyed and may move on and kill additional targets. T cells of this kind develop with specificities against antigens on cells in grafted tissues and they are important in the rejection of such grafts.

Until recently this type of immunity was considered to be mediated only by T lymphocytes, but it would now appear that other cell types play a part:

1. *Natural killer cells (NK cells)*—These cells are capable non-specifically of killing tumour cells or virally infected cells.
2. *Killer cells (K cells)*—Although also part of the non-specific immune system these cells, unlike NK cells, can only kill target cells when they are coated with antibody. However, they recognize the Fc end of the molecule, not the antibody-combining site. They are also known as *antibody-dependent cytotoxic cells* (ADCC).
3. *Macrophages*—important in the processing of antigen to both B and T lymphocytes. Moreover, they may take part directly in the destruction of target cells by phagocytosis and by direct cytotoxic effects on antibody-coated target cells in a manner similar to K cells.

Both NK and K cells look like large lymphocytes; however, their origin is not yet known. Together they are sometimes referred to as '*null cells*'.

Examples of lymphokines and their activities

1. Affecting other lymphocytes
Interferons
Interleukin-2
B cell growth and differentiation factors
Assorted helper and suppressor factors

2. Affecting macrophages
Chemotactic factor
Migration inhibition factor
Activation factor

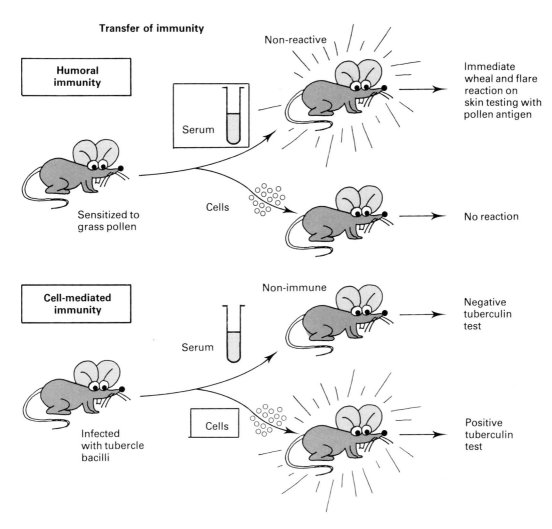

Transfer of immunity

Humoral immunity

Serum

Sensitized to grass pollen

Cells

Non-reactive

Immediate wheal and flare reaction on skin testing with pollen antigen

No reaction

Cell-mediated immunity

Serum

Infected with tubercle bacilli

Cells

Non-immune

Negative tuberculin test

Positive tuberculin test

Some differences between humoral immunity and cell-mediated immunity

There are two fundamental distinctions between humoral and cell-mediated immune responses *in vivo*:

1. *Rate of response*.
2. *Method of transfer*.

Rate of response

An example of a humoral response is the *immediate* wheal and flare reaction which occurs about 15 minutes after an extract of grass pollen antigen is injected into the skin of a person with hay fever or asthma caused by grass pollen. In contrast, an example of a cell-mediated reaction is the *delayed* hypersensitivity response seen in the *tuberculin test*. This reaction occurs when a small amount of antigen from tubercle bacilli is injected under the skin of an individual previously sensitized to the antigen, and consists of an area of erythema and induration occurring 24–48 hours after injection.

Method of transfer

The ability to produce both humoral and cell-mediated responses to an antigen can be transferred from an immune individual to a non-immune individual, but the method of acquisition is different in each case. Humoral responses, e.g. the ability to give an immediate wheal and flare reaction, can be transferred to a normal person with *serum* from a hypersensitive person. However, immunity to tuberculosis cannot be transferred in this way. It is necessary to transfer *lymphoid cells*. Similarly, the ability to reject tissue grafts can be transferred with cells but not usually with serum.

Genetic control of the immune response

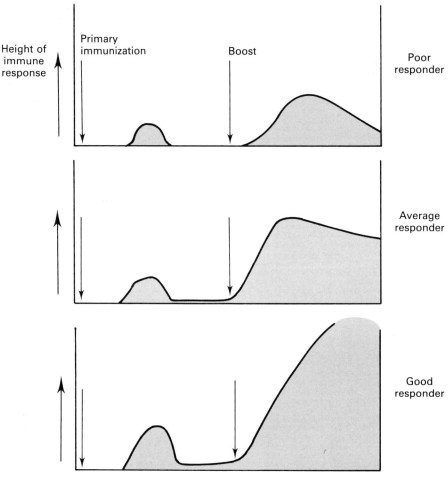

Height of immune response

Primary immunization

Boost

Poor responder

Average responder

Good responder

Our genes dictate to a large degree whether we are tall or small, intelligent or dim-witted, etc.

It appears that they also play a major part in determining whether we will make good or poor responses to various antigens

10. Control of the immune response

When a humoral immune response is initiated by antigen a *feedback mechanism* operates to dampen it down, i.e. as antibody levels increase, excess antigen is 'mopped up', leaving less available to act as an antigenic stimulus.

However, the overall control of the immune system is much more complex and as yet is not fully understood. There are several levels of regulation: A. *genetic*, B. *cellular* and C. *molecular*.

A. Genetic control

Some species are better than others at producing antibody against certain kinds of antigen. For example, rabbits usually produce high levels of antibody to soluble proteins, while mice respond poorly to such antigens. Moreover, within species it has been found that some genetic types are good antibody producers, while others are bad—*responders* and *non-responders*.

It is now clear that a number of specific immune response (Ir) genes exist which control specific responses and are in close association with genes coding for the major histocompatibility antigens (see p. 81).

Cellular control of the immune response

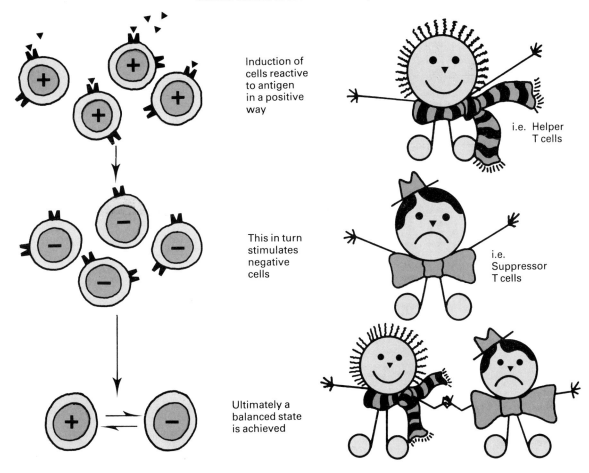

Induction of cells reactive to antigen in a positive way

This in turn stimulates negative cells

Ultimately a balanced state is achieved

i.e. Helper T cells

i.e. Suppressor T cells

B. Cellular control

The specific immune response is classically divided into two branches: the antibody-mediated immunity of B lymphocytes, and the cell-mediated immunity of T lymphocytes.

However, T cells also play an important role in regulating the production of antibodies by B cells. T–B cell cooperation is necessary for antibody production to take place. There are two main types of T lymphocytes that appear to be important in the regulation of the immune response: *helper* and *suppressor* T cells. *Helper T cells*, on interaction with an antigenic molecule, release substances which help B lymphocytes to produce antibodies against this antigen.

Suppressor T cells, it is thought, can 'turn off' B cells so that they can no longer cooperate with normal T cells to induce an immune response.

The normal immune response probably represents a very fine balance between the action of *helper* and *suppressor* T cells. It is possible that many clinical conditions may result from an upset in this balance. For example:

1. It has been shown that patients with some types of immunoglobulin deficiency have an increase in suppressor cell activity.
2. It has been suggested that there is an enhancement of suppressor cell function in patients with multiple myeloma. The normal polyclonal antibody response of the myeloma patient may be suppressed by these cells, with an increased susceptibility to infection resulting.
3. There is evidence to indicate that suppressor cells are closely involved in the control of autoimmune disease. It is thought that with advancing age there is a decrease in number or function of suppressor T cells which allows for the production of autoantibodies.

In addition to modulating the B cell response, suppressor T cells also appear to regulate the activities of other T cells.

C. Molecular control

(i) The interleukins

Various soluble substances are produced from cells of the immune system. If they are produced from activated lymphocytes they can be classified as *lymphokines*. However, cells other than lymphocytes can produce soluble products which have effects on other cells. These substances can almost be regarded as the means by which cells 'speak to each other' and 'direct' each other into particular activities.

The *interleukins* are an example of such substances and their overall effect is to 'switch on' and augment the immune response of T lymphocytes. Their activity therefore can be considered to be part of the regulatory system.

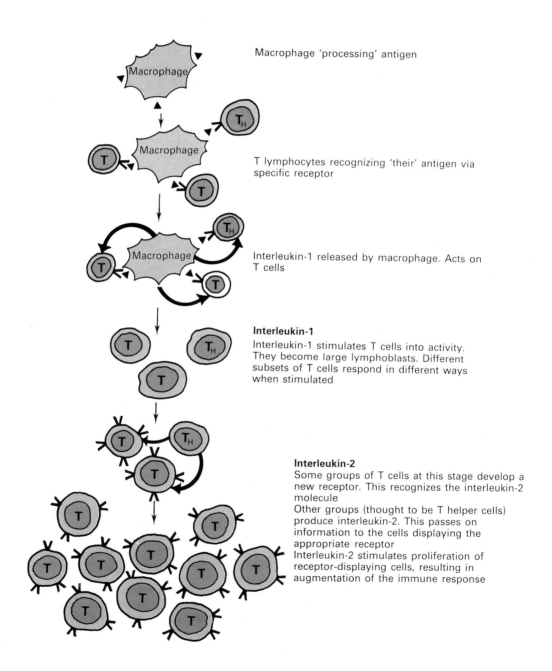

Macrophage 'processing' antigen

T lymphocytes recognizing 'their' antigen via specific receptor

Interleukin-1 released by macrophage. Acts on T cells

Interleukin-1

Interleukin-1 stimulates T cells into activity. They become large lymphoblasts. Different subsets of T cells respond in different ways when stimulated

Interleukin-2

Some groups of T cells at this stage develop a new receptor. This recognizes the interleukin-2 molecule

Other groups (thought to be T helper cells) produce interleukin-2. This passes on information to the cells displaying the appropriate receptor

Interleukin-2 stimulates proliferation of receptor-displaying cells, resulting in augmentation of the immune response

(ii) Jerne's network theory

It is thought that a sophisticated network of antibody production between the components of the immune system exists and that this functions as an extremely important part of the regulatory system. As a result, fine control is achieved, some parts being switched off while others are switched on. It is a fairly complicated theory, but the diagrams below illustrate the main points. The theory has not yet been fully confirmed experimentally.

First of all it is important to understand what is meant by the term *idiotype*.

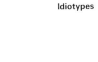

Idiotypes

The variable regions of an antibody molecule make up the *idiotypic structure* of that molecule

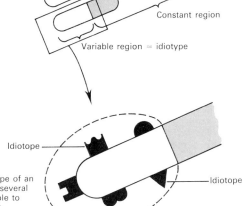

Constant region

Variable region = idiotype

Like an antigen, however, the idiotype of an immunoglobulin molecule contains several *antigenic determinants*, each one able to initiate a different immune response
Each of the antigenic determinants is called an *idiotope*

Idiotope

Idiotope

Idiotope

The network theory postulates that *autoantibodies to idiotopes* are produced during the normal immune response. These are known as *anti-idiotype antibodies*

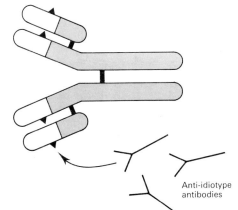

Anti-idiotype antibodies

Cells displaying idiotype structures

The importance of anti-idiotype antibodies is not their effect on freely circulating immunoglobulin molecules but rather their effect on cells

As previously mentioned (p.32), B cells have a receptor (membrane-bound immunoglobulin) and T cells a different but similar receptor. Both receptors display the specific chemical structure similar to the antibody end of an immunoglobulin molecule, i.e. they both display their own highly specific idiotypes

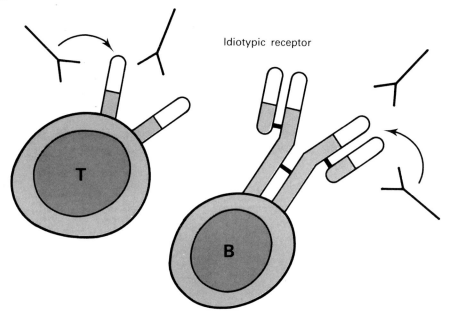

Idiotypic receptor

The effect of anti-idiotype antibodies

It is likely that the binding of some anti-idiotype immunoglobulins to cells has the effect of switching off the immune response and others have an opposite stimulatory effect

Anti-anti-idiotype antibodies

To make matters even more complicated, it appears that yet other groups of lymphocytes can make antibody to the anti-idiotype immunoglobulin. Hence a network of interactions is thought to take place—the net result of which is thought to be the exquisitely sensitive regulation of the immune response

If Jerne's network theory turns out to be true, there are implications that 'immunization' using highly specific anti–idiotype antibodies could modify the immune response in graft rejection, autoimmunity and some types of hypersensitivity state. Such intervention will undoubtedly prove very difficult and even if possible is a long way off.

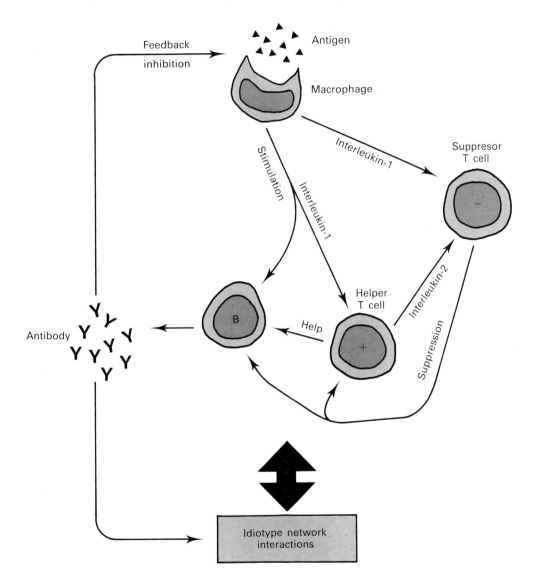

An overview of immunoregulation

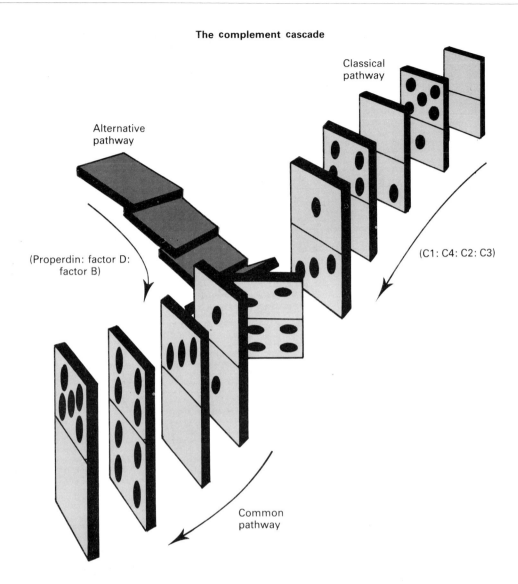

The complement cascade

Classical
pathway

Alternative
pathway

(Properdin: factor D:
factor B)

(C1: C4: C2: C3)

Common
pathway

11. The complement system

The *complement system* is a complex enzymatic system composed of a series of proteins which interact sequentially with one another in a 'cascade' fashion. The system reacts like a line of dominoes—when the first member is activated it triggers off all the succeeding members.

The complement system performs two basic functions:

1. It is an essential part of the body's defence against bacteria and viruses. Hereditary complement deficiencies in man are frequently associated with recurrent infections.
2. It is involved in the inflammatory process and in the mediation of immunological tissue injury,

Complement activation follows either the *classical* or the *alternative pathway*, but both converge on C3, the keystone of the system.

The classical pathway

The classical pathway functions in three distinct phases:

1. The '*recognition unit*' (C1q, C1r, C1s).
2. The '*activation unit*' (C4, C2, C3) (N.B. The sequence of classical activation is C1→C4→C2→C3 *not* C1→C2→C3→C4).
3. The '*membrane attack unit*' (C5, C6, C7, C8, C9).

The complement components found in the serum are the building blocks from which these three elements are assembled following activation. Activation of this pathway is by immune complexes formed by IgM and IgG antibodies.

The alternative pathway

The alternative pathway consists of at least three distinct proteins—properdin, factor D, and factor B. The end result is an enzyme which activates C3 and the remainder of the complement sequence. In effect, the alternative pathway bypasses C1, C4 and C2 of the classical pathway. Activation of this pathway can be initiated by aggregated immunoglobulins IgG, IgA, and IgE. In addition, the alternative pathway may be triggered by bacterial endotoxins (bacterial cell walls), and zymosan (yeast cell walls). Therefore, certain of the complement-mediated defence effects can take place before the appearance of specific antibody.

Dynamics

In general, the activation of the components of the complement system involves enzymatic cleavage of each component into two fragments. The larger of the two fragments joins the activated preceding component, thus generating a new enzymatic activity which is capable of cleaving the next component. The smaller fragments in the earlier stages frequently have important inflammatory properties of their own.

Once activated, the complement sequence does not continue to cascade. Regulation is achieved by the natural instability and short active life of some of the activated components, and by serum inhibitors such as C1 inhibitor, C3b inactivator, C6 inactivator, and anaphylatoxin inactivator.

Role of complement in defence

Complement mediates the attack on invading microorganisms. The function of antibody is to identify the invading organism as foreign and to activate the attack of complement. Once activated, the complement system sets in motion a series of processes that destroy the foreign cell.

A. *Cell lysis*

The full complement system leading to membrane damage can cause the destruction of some bacteria by rupture so that the cells release their contents.

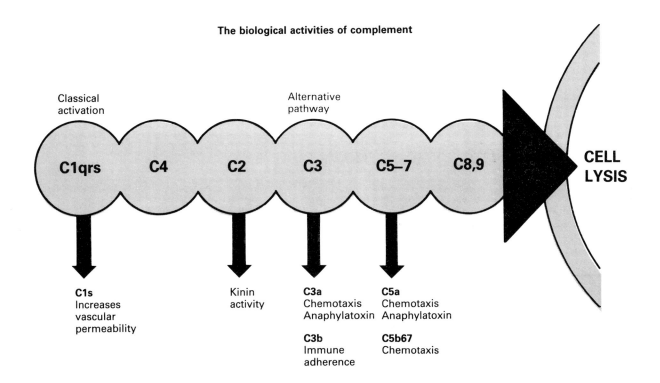

The biological activities of complement

Cytotoxic effect of complement

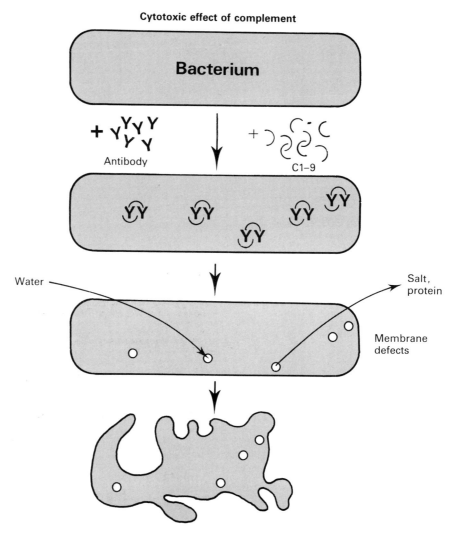

B. *Promotion of phagocytosis*

This is achieved by two mechanisms.

1. *Opsonization*—activated C3 molecules bind to microorganisms. Neutrophils and macrophages have specific binding sites for C3b thus facilitating phagocytosis of the coated organisms.
2. *Inflammation*—the movement, i.e. *chemotaxis*, of phagocytic cells towards the microorganism and the *increase in vascular permeability* that is seen as a feature of acute inflammation are promoted by the release of small fragments of complement components during the course of activation.

Role of complement in disease

In some individuals the control of complement is not perfect and damage may be done to the host's own cells. Complement plays a major role in the pathogenesis of immune complex disease. For example, in systemic lupus erythematosus, the interaction of DNA and anti-DNA results in complement activation and the production of inflammatory factors (*anaphylotoxins*) at sites where complexes have been lodged. If this occurs in renal glomeruli or in the walls of blood vessels, the result is immunological injury. If, by accident, the body makes antibody to its own red cells, the complement system has no way of distinguishing the coated red cells from any other foreign cells. The interaction of complement with antigen–antibody complexes on the cell surface leads to the destruction of red cells.

On the one hand, complement aids immune protection; on the other hand, it contributes to hypersensitivity and autoimmune disorders.

Section B
Clinical conditions involving immunological mechanisms

Gell and Coombs' classification of hypersensitivity mechanisms

Type I	Antibody-mediated Also known as immediate hypersensitivity, anaphylactic or IgE-mediated

Type II	Antibody-mediated Also known as cytotoxic hypersensitivity

Type III	Antibody-mediated Also known as immune-complex hypersensitivity

Type IV	Cell-mediated Also known as delayed-type hypersensitivity

12. Hypersensitivity

Hypersensitivity—some terminology

The immune response, when it 'goes wrong', can cause a whole spectrum of disease states affecting any of the organs of the body. As with any other immune reaction, the individual must first have become 'sensitized' by previous exposure to the antigen. On second and subsequent exposures, symptoms and signs of a hypersensitivity state can occur *immediately* or be *delayed* until several days later. The terms *immediate* and *delayed*, however, have changed their meaning over the years. Nowadays, *immediate hypersensitivity* refers to *antibody-mediated* reactions, while *delayed hypersensitivity* refers to *cell-mediated* reactions.

Hypersensitivity—
This denotes a state of *increased reactivity* of the host to an antigen and implies that the reaction is damaging to the host. The increased reactivity which, for example, follows immunization procedures is beneficial and is not described as a hypersensitive state.

Allergy—
In modern usage allergy is synonymous with *hypersensitivity*. The antigen capable of eliciting an allergic or hypersensitive state is known as an *allergen*. *Anergic* means the opposite of allergic, i.e. the individual shows no immune response to an antigen that he has met previously.

More than twenty years ago, an attempt was made to classify these hypersensitivity reactions according to the underlying immune mechanisms involved. Four types of hypersensitive states were described and this classification is still loosely accepted today, although it is becoming clear that there is considerable overlap in the mechanisms involved.

The symptoms of atopy

Anaphylaxis*
Asthma
Eczema
Hay fever
Allergic conjunctivitis
Urticaria
Gastrointestinal symptoms

*Anaphylaxis is rare. All the other symptoms are much commoner. It is placed top of the list because it is by far the most serious manifestation.

Type I (immediate) hypersensitivity

About 10% of the people reading this page dread the time of year when the pollen count is high because it brings on their *hay fever*. On the other hand, they may have been troubled from childhood with *eczema* or, worse still, be prone to *asthmatic attacks*. These are the people who are described as *atopic*. *Atopy* means strangeness and describes the 'strange', formerly poorly understood, reactions that these individuals appear to have to common substances. It is now known that atopy is due to abnormal and inappropriate IgE production. IgE is probably important in the protection against parasitic disease; however, in Britain at least, it appears to do more harm than good. When an atopic individual meets common substances such as grass pollen, house dust, or house dust mite, IgE rather than the more usual IgG class of antibodies are produced. These antibodies have an affinity for *mast cells* or *basophils* and attach to them. This in itself is harmless until the IgE meets up with its specific allergen. Immediately this happens the *mast cell* is triggered to discharge its contents of *vasoactive subtances* into the circulation. This release leads to the symptoms of sneezing, running nose, red watery eyes, and perhaps wheezing. When the allergen is removed the symptoms subside even although specific IgE antibody remains bound to mast cells.

Type I hypersensitivity is probably the commonest immunological abnormality seen in medical practice. Fortunately, however, although as many as 10% of the population are atopic, most of these people suffer from irritating rather than serious symptoms.

Examples of the type of allergens responsible for atopic symptoms

House dust mite
Pollens
Animal danders, e.g. cat, dog, horse
Foods, e.g. milk, egg, peanuts
Moulds, e.g. *Aspergillus*
Animal serum, e.g. horse serum previously used in
    some vaccines

Drugs*

*Many drugs function as *haptens* rather than true allergens or antigens, i.e. they are low molecular weight substances which cannot produce an immune response on their own. However, when they combine with tissue or serum proteins, the hapten–protein complex *can* elicit an immune response specific for the antigenic determinants of the hapten. This immune response *may* involve IgE mechanisms.

Mechanisms involved in type I hypersensitivity

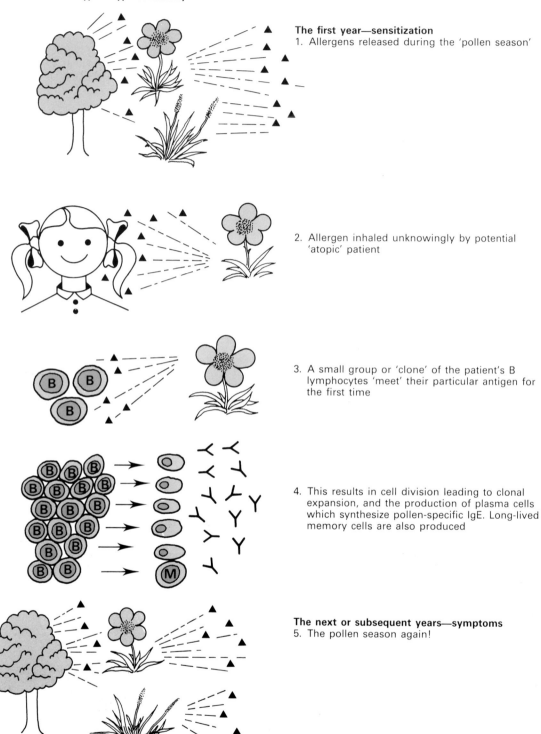

The first year—sensitization
1. Allergens released during the 'pollen season'

2. Allergen inhaled unknowingly by potential 'atopic' patient

3. A small group or 'clone' of the patient's B lymphocytes 'meet' their particular antigen for the first time

4. This results in cell division leading to clonal expansion, and the production of plasma cells which synthesize pollen-specific IgE. Long-lived memory cells are also produced

The next or subsequent years—symptoms
5. The pollen season again!

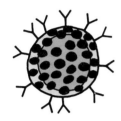

6. Specific IgE antibody produced much earlier and in much larger amounts owing to immunological memory

7. The Fc end of the IgE molecule binds to tissue mast cells and circulating basophils

Cross-linking antigen

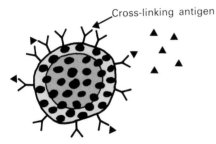

8. If the patient is still exposed to the pollen, these molecules will bind to the Fab end of the IgE molecule

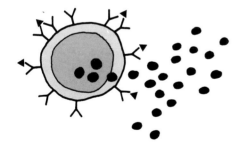

9. If antigen cross-links two specific IgE molecules, the cell is triggered to release the granules into the circulation. These granules contain certain substances, such as histamine, which have far-reaching effects on organs throughout the body

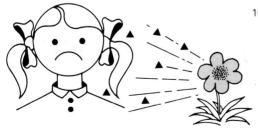

10. Symptoms develop
In the case of pollen allergy as described symptoms generally take the form of rhino-conjunctivitis or sometimes asthma
In the case of an allergen which is present throughout the year, e.g. house dust mite, symptoms are perennial

Anaphylaxis

This is the most serious and fortunately very rare symptom of the atopic state. The symptoms are related totally to the massive release of vasoactive substances leading to fall in blood pressure, shock, difficulty in breathing and even death. Anaphylaxis can be the result of, for example, a bee sting, a penicillin injection, an injection of horse serum (e.g. formerly used in protection against tetanus), in a previously sensitized person.

Several decades ago the use of horse serum for vaccine purposes was widespread and this was the commonest cause of anaphylaxis. Now we have the antibiotic era with its consequences. Penicillin in particular has become the most common cause of death due to anaphylaxis. This is much more likely after parenteral administration of the drug. it is extremely important that every patient who is to receive penicillin or a related antibiotic is asked carefully about previous penicillin reactions BEFORE it is administered.

One would expect that, since IgE mechanisms are responsible for true anaphylaxis it would only occur in patients who have previously demonstrated clinical symptoms of atopy. This is not necessarily the case. Research in this area is difficult, however, because of the rarity of the condition.

Clinical features

Symptoms of anaphlaxis can occur immediately, i.e. within a few seconds of exposure to the antigen or hapten to which the patient is sensitive. However, reactions can also appear as long as one hour after exposure.

Usually many systems of the body are involved simultaneously, i.e. the cardiovascular system, the respiratory tract, the skin and the gastrointestinal tract. Sometimes, however, only one system is involved.

Clinical features of anaphylaxis

General symptoms

Feeling of warmth*
Light-headedness*
Feeling of impending doom

Respiratory tract

Hoarseness of voice	Oedema of epiglottis and
Stridor	larynx can cause fatal upper
Lump in the throat	airways obstruction
Shortness of breath	Severe asthmatic attack with
Tightness in chest	associated lack of oxygen
Wheezing	can follow

Cardiovascular system

Hypotension
Acute myocardial ischaemia
Cardiac arrhythmias

Skin

Skin erythema, pruritus
Urticaria
Angioedema

Gastrointestinal tract
Nausea
Vomiting
Abdominal pain
Tenesmus
Haematemesis
Diarrhoea

Uterus
Uterine cramps

---

*Remember—A simple vaso-vagal attack (faint) is much more common after an injection than anaphylaxis.

Treatment and prevention of anaphylaxis

Early recognition of the condition and early administration of adrenaline are considered essential. Other drugs which may be of benefit are aminophylline, antihistamines, and steroids.

It is sometimes advocated that a tourniquet be used to decrease exposure to a parenterally administered substance. For example, if the patient was exposed to a bee sting on the lower leg, a tourniquet could be applied to the thigh. Great care must be taken, however, that the blood flow to the extremity is not impaired by such measures.

Above all, very close observation is necessary. An intravenous line should be inserted, and pulse, respiration and blood pressure should be frequently charted. Arterial blood pH, pO_2 and pCO_2 should be assayed and a cardiac monitor should be attached to detect myocardial ischaemia and arrythmias. Endotracheal intubation should be performed sooner rather than later if severe respiratory obstruction becomes evident. Full resuscitative measures may be necessary in spite of early diagnosis and treatment.

Any patient who has had an anaphylactic reaction, even if treated adequately and apparently making excellent recovery, should be kept in hospital overnight and observed closely.

Prevention is of course better than cure and it is essential that all patients should be fully questioned regarding allergic reactions as a routine part of their medical history. They should be questioned again prior to the administration of substances known to be associated with anaphylaxis. However, even with the best will in the world, anaphylaxis more often occurs unexpectedly in a patient who has had a previous uneventful exposure. It is essential therefore that all medical and nursing staff are always aware of and recognize the unexpected.

Treatment of anaphylaxis

TREAT IMMEDIATELY AND ENSURE AN ADEQUATE AIRWAY THROUGHOUT

1. Lay patient down

2. Give 0.5 ml 1:1000 adrenaline injection BP intramuscularly close to injection site. Repeat to a total of 2 ml over a 15-minute period

3. If bronchospasm is still present in spite of adrenaline, give 10–20 ml aminophylline BP (250 mg/10 ml) SLOWLY intravenously (no faster than 2 ml per minute)

4. 200–400 mg hydrocortisone injection BP should be given intravenously. This may help prevent late reactions such as bronchospasm

5. Monitor the patient's clinical state throughout and use full supportive measures if necessary

6. Observe patient closely for at least 24 hours

7. Warn patient against future reactions and supply him with a warning card or bracelet

(N.B. The doses above refer to the adult patient. They should be modified appropriately in the child.)

Anaphylactoid reactions

Sometimes features identical to anaphylaxis are seen but there is no evidence that IgE-mediated hypersensitivity plays a part in the mechanism. Such reactions are known as anaphylactoid.

One of the most common causes of a non-IgE-mediated anaphylactoid reaction is that observed in about 1% of the population following the intravenous administration of RADIOCONTRAST MEDIA. Because of the relatively high frequency of such reactions, adrenaline and other resuscitative measures should always be at hand when such media are injected in X-ray departments. The underlying immunological mechanism may result from activation of complement by the contrast medium. Vasoactive substances are probably produced which exert widespread effects. These substances, however, have not yet been identified.

Some commonly used drugs, e.g. morphine, are capable of *directly* causing degranulation of mast cells with no evidence of IgE involvement.

Occasionally, physical factors such as cold water immersion or strenuous exercise can induce anaphylactoid reactions.

Immunotherapy

This type of therapy is also known as hyposensitization or desensitization.

It involves giving a course of subcutaneous injections of gradually increasing strengths of extracts of allergen to which the patient is known to be sensitive. Such therapy has in some patients been shown to decrease their symptoms on future exposure.

The mechanisms involved in desensitization are not yet fully understood and the results are unpredictable.

There is always a small risk of a serious anaphylactic reaction during desensitization so the possible benefits of the procedure must be carefully weighed against the risks. The technique should be done in a hospital environment where full resuscitative equipment and expertise are at hand.

Type II (cytotoxic) hypersensitivity

This type of allergic reaction occurs when circulating antibody combines directly with host tissues which for some reason are recognized as foreign. This may be due to a cross-reacting antibody or may be the result of antigens or haptens bound to the cell wall. Once antibody binds, other mechanisms such as complement activation and damage by neutrophils leads to destruction of the target cells.

Well-known common examples of this type of hypersensitivity are *transfusion reactions* due to mismatched blood or *Rhesus incompatibility*. A less common example is *Goodpasture's syndrome*, where the patient develops pulmonary and renal symptoms due to a cross-reacting antibody with lung and renal tissue.

Transfusion reactions

An individual's red blood cells carry several types of antigens. The best known of these antigenic systems is the ABO.

The basis of this is as follows:

Blood group A

If an individual is blood group A, this means his red blood cells carry antigen A. The individual would not normally make antibodies to A or he would haemolyse his own red blood cells and become very anaemic: his own A antigen is recognized as 'self' and is 'tolerated', i.e. no immune response appears to be mounted against it. Such an individual, however, has no B antigen on his red cells. One would expect, if exposed to another person's blood cells which express the B antigen, that he would recognize these as foreign and make antibody to them. Previous exposure to foreign cells is not necessary in order to sensitize the patient because for some reason naturally occuring antibodies to this system occur. This is thought to be due to cross-reactivity with very similar antigenic determinants on microorganisms colonizing the individual early in life.

Blood group B

The red cells of such an individual express the B antigen. There is *no* anti-B in the serum but antibody to A *is* present since this is recognized as foreign.

Blood group AB

These cells express BOTH A and B antigens. Both are recognized as self and so no antibodies to A or B are present in the serum.

Blood group O

Individuals with blood group O express NEITHER A nor B antigens on their red blood cells and so antibody to BOTH antigens is found in the serum. In Britain O and A are the commonest blood groups. Groups B and AB are uncommon.

A mismatched blood transfusion implies that the recipient's serum contains antibody to the donor red cells. This would happen if for example cells expressing A antigen were transfused into a patient of blood group B. Such a patient would have antibody to A and as a result destruction of the donor cells would take place. Transfusion reactions are characterized by one or more of the symptoms in the accompanying diagram.

The ABO blood group system

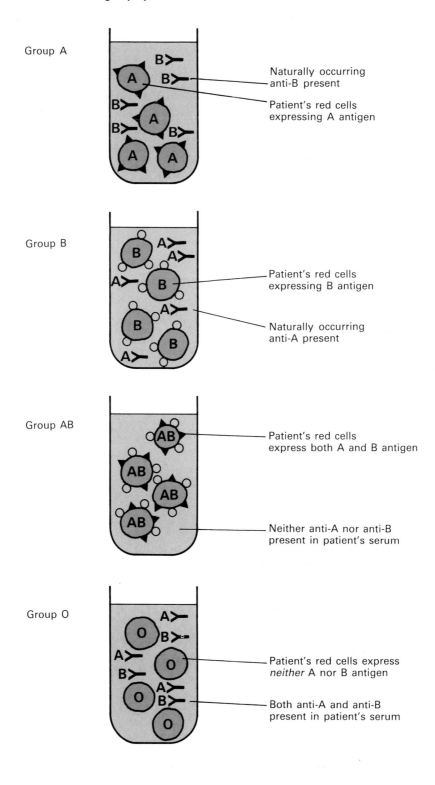

Group A

Naturally occurring anti-B present

Patient's red cells expressing A antigen

Group B

Patient's red cells expressing B antigen

Naturally occurring anti-A present

Group AB

Patient's red cells express both A and B antigen

Neither anti-A nor anti-B present in patient's serum

Group O

Patient's red cells express *neither* A nor B antigen

Both anti-A and anti-B present in patient's serum

The consequences of a mismatched tranfusion

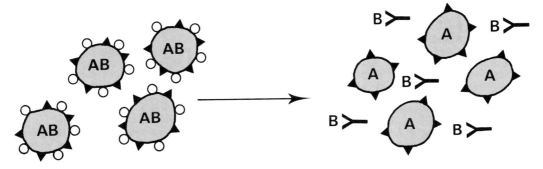

Donor cells

Recipient's cells
and antibody

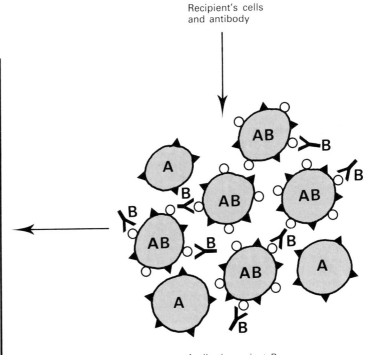

Antibody against B
binds to target cell.
Complement is activated
and the cell ruptured

Symptoms of a
transfusion reaction

- Fever
- Shock
- Chest tightness
- Gastrointestinal symptoms
- Haemolysis
- Anaemia
- Jaundice

Immune complex formation — a normal event

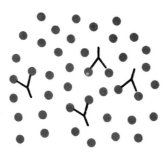

Immune complexes formed
in antigen excess

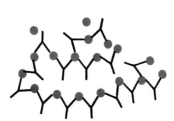

Immune complexes formed
in equivalence

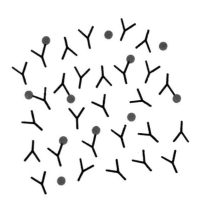

Immune complexes formed
in antibody excess

but
Many antigen/antibody ratios are possible

Type III (immune complex-mediated) hypersensitivity

During the normal immune response, antibody is of course produced as a result of exposure to antigen. At some time during this response *immune complexes* composed of varying proportions of antigen and antibody are produced. It is likely that all of us from time to time have circulating immune complexes (e.g. during the course of infectious diseases). Mostly they cause no symptoms and quickly disappear from the circulation.

In some individuals, however, immune complexes can persist in the circulation and may cause clinical symptoms, some of them serious. The size of the complexes produced seems important in determining whether they will be eliminated quickly from the body or retained long enough to cause damage.

The classical clinical symptoms of immune complex disease are due to blood vessel involvement,

i.e. *vasculitis*. The blood vessels of joints and the kidneys are most frequently affected, giving rise to symptoms and signs of *arthritis* and *glomerulonephritis*.

The mechanisms of type III hypersensitivity are as follows:

1. *Soluble* immune complexes which contain a greater proportion of antigen than antibody penetrate blood vessels and lodge on the *basement membrane*. (Complexes that are larger and insoluble are easily removed by polymorphs and macrophages and do no harm.)
2. At the basement membrane site, these complexes activate the *complement cascade*.
3. During complement activation, certain products of the cascade are produced. These are able to

Pathological immune complexes

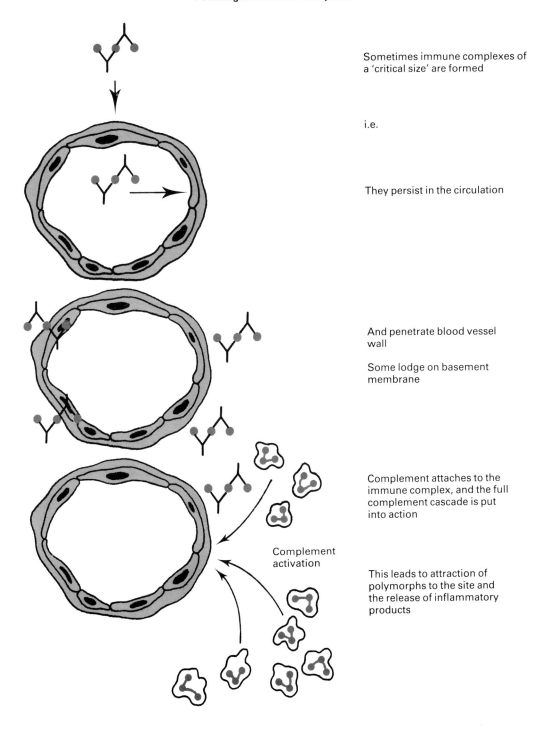

Sometimes immune complexes of a 'critical size' are formed

i.e.

They persist in the circulation

And penetrate blood vessel wall

Some lodge on basement membrane

Complement attaches to the immune complex, and the full complement cascade is put into action

Complement activation

This leads to attraction of polymorphs to the site and the release of inflammatory products

Animal model of immune complex disease

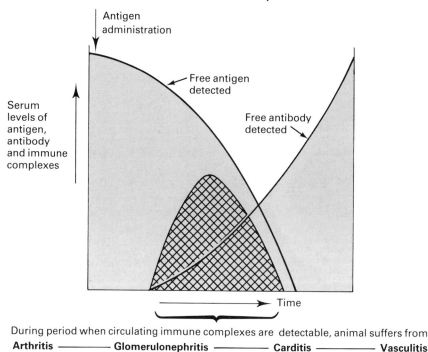

Serum
levels of
antigen,
antibody
and immune
complexes

Antigen
administration

Free antigen
detected

Free antibody
detected

Time

During period when circulating immune complexes are detectable, animal suffers from

Arthritis ———— Glomerulonephritis ———— Carditis ———— Vasculitis

attract *neutrophils* to the area. Such substances are known as *chemotactic substances*.

4. Once the neutrophils reach the basement membrane they release their granules, which contain *lysosomal enzymes*. These enzymes are damaging to the blood vessels.

This total process leads to the condition recognized histologically as *vasculitis*.

When a type III hypersensitivity reaction occurs *locally* (e.g. in the skin), it is known as an *Arthus reaction*. When it occurs *systemically*, i.e. as a result of *circulating* immune complexes, it is known as *serum sickness*.

The symptoms of serum sickness were recognized early in the twentieth century, when foreign serum was administered to patients for the purpose of protecting them from an infectious disease. Such a procedure is seldom used nowadays. However, type III hypersensitivity is undoubtedly the mechanism involved in many other conditions. For example:

1. *Streptococcal disease*—Immune complexes of streptococcal antigens and their specific antibodies are a well-known cause of glomerulonephritis.

2. *Disseminated lupus erythematosus.* In this autoimmune disease antibody is made against the patient's own DNA. DNA–anti-DNA complexes circulate and lead to the symptoms of arthritis and glomerulonephritis so common in this condition.

3. *Farmer's lung* is one cause of the condition known as *extrinsic allergic alveolitis*. These patients suffer from fever, cough and breathlessness after exposure to mouldy hay. This is because one of the microorganisms residing in mouldy hay is inhaled and the farmer, for example, who has already produced antibody to it develops a local type III hypersensitivity state leading to vasculitis in the lungs.

4. *Miscellaneous conditions.* Many infections such as hepatitis, malaria, syphilis, and glandular fever, have from time to time been recorded as being associated with circulating immune complex disease.

In the human, immune complex disease can be no more than a transient minor inconvenience leading to mild symptoms of arthralgia. However, at the other extreme, it can lead to widespread, severe, life-threatening disease. When this stage is reached we often use immunosuppressive therapy to 'dampen down' the immune response.

One of the great challenges in immunology for the future is to learn how to manipulate the specific immune response in such a way that immune complexes of a 'dangerous' size and configuration are not made. The other important area is that we try to identify the antigens involved, so that if possible, at least in some cases, patients can be kept away from offending substances.

Tuberculous granuloma

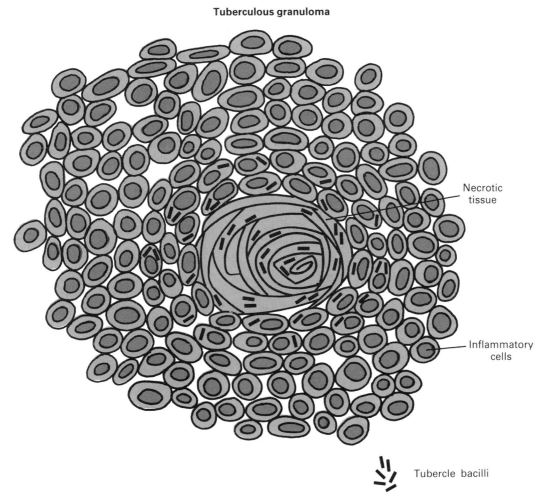

Necrotic tissue

Inflammatory cells

Tubercle bacilli

Type IV (delayed) hypersensitivity

The terms type IV hypersensitivity or *delayed hypersensitivity* are used to describe the symptoms and signs associated with a *cell-mediated* immune response.

Unlike the types of hypersensitivity state previously discussed, antibody and complement are not involved in type IV responses. It is purely a result of reactions involving *T lymphocytes*. Another difference is in the time interval between exposure and response. Type IV reactions occur about two days following antigenic exposure, whereas reactions involving antibody occur within minutes or a few hours.

Certain conditions are known to be associated with cell-mediated reactions which are damaging to the host. Sometimes there is a fairly fine balance between protective and damaging effects, for example, during the course of tuberculosis *granulomata* are formed. These lesions represent the body's cell-mediated response to the tubercle bacillus. As a result, the organism is effectively 'walled-off' from the rest of the body and is unable to disseminate and do further damage. However, the large caseating lung abscesses in tuberculosis can be regarded as an effect of the body's immune response to the organism rather than direct damage by the organism itself. In some situations the 'balance' is tipped totally against the host, i.e. cell-mediated reactions in certain circumstances are wholly damaging, with no apparent beneficial effect at all. This is seen in the following conditions:

1. *Drug allergy and allergic response to insect bites and 'stings'.* Type I and type III responses are often also involved in these 'allergies'. Sometimes, however,

a type IV response is responsible, or it may contribute to a coexisting type I or type III response.

2. *Contact dermatitis.* Eczema or dermatitis can either be part of a type I 'atopic' state or involve a cell-mediated hypersensitivity reaction. Eczema associated with a cell-mediated reaction is usually described as '*contact dermatitis*' because, in general, direct contact between skin and the offending agent is necessary before hypersensitivity results. This is not the case in most eczemas due to type I allergy.

Many common substances such as *metals*, *paints*, *cosmetics* and *plants* have been implicated in these reactions. The reaction only occurs, of course, on second or subsequent exposure to the substance(s) after sensitization has taken place. However, in many cases, the individual has been exposed over many years to the offending substance without any harmful effects and a delayed hypersensitivity reactions appears 'out of the blue'. Because of this patients sometimes find it difficult to believe they can possibly be allergic to familiar substances.

Very often the lesions affect only that area of the skin in contact with the offending agent, but this is not necessarily the case. For example, a woman who is allergic to nickel may develop severe widespread dermatitis as a result of wearing gold ear-rings. This is because even jewellery made from precious metals contains a little nickel. The patient in this situation would find it hard to believe her ear-rings were responsible for such severe symptoms.

3. *Rejection of grafts.* Graft rejection is predominantly a cell-mediated function, and of course in the organ transplant situation is very detrimental to the host.

4. *Autoimmune diseases.* Some autoimmune diseases seem to be the result of a type IV hypersensitivity state. This is discussed in more detail in chapter 14.

Examples of delayed hypersensitivity reactions that are detrimental to the host

Drug allergy

Allergic response to insect bites and stings

Contact dermatitis

Rejection of grafts

Some autoimmune diseases

Classification of immunodeficiency

Immunodeficiency can be classified in two ways:
   A. According to whether it is primary or secondary.
   B. According to which limbs of the immune system are affected.

Classification A	Classification B
SECONDARY	Defect of non-specific immune system
1. Much more common than primary immune deficiency	
2. Occurs during the course of many medical conditions, often directly as a result of treatment	Defect of humoral immunity
3. There may be an underlying viral infection (e.g. AIDS)	Defect of cell-mediated immunity
PRIMARY	or
1. Many are very rare conditions	
2. There is no apparent underlying medical condition	More than one limb of the immune response may be involved
3. No immunosuppressive therapy has been given	
4. There is no known underlying viral infection	

(N.B. Secondary immunodeficiency is considered before primary immunodeficiency. This is to emphasize the fact that secondary immunodeficiencies are much more common.)

13. Immunodeficiency

The symptoms of immunodeficiency

The cardinal symptom of immunodeficiency is *infection*—recurrent, severe, or presenting in an unusual way. This may involve the skin, mucous membranes, lungs or gastrointestinal tract. It may present as a life-threatening condition such as meningitis or septicaemia. Although patients with immunodeficiency suffer from infections due to all the 'normal' pathogens, they are, in addition, liable to infection with organisms normally considered to be of low pathogenicity.

In general, deficiencies of the non-specific and humoral immune systems are associated with *bacterial infections*, whereas deficiencies of the cell-mediated limb are associated with *viral, fungal, protozoal* or *mycobacterial infections*.

It is important to remember, however, that in spite of antibiotics and immunization, infections occur very frequently in 'normal' individuals. Recurrent infections are also symptomatic of many underlying medical conditions such as diabetes and fibrocystic disease, and such conditions should always first be excluded before embarking on a full investigation of a patient's immune function.

Some examples of simple hospital procedures which compromise the host

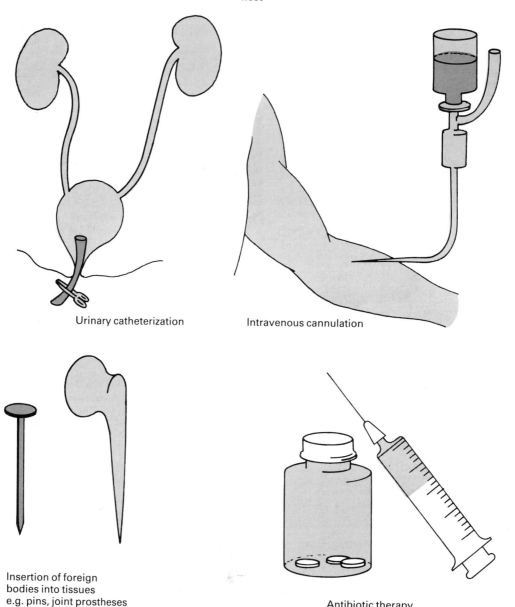

Urinary catheterization

Intravenous cannulation

Insertion of foreign
bodies into tissues
e.g. pins, joint prostheses

Antibiotic therapy

Secondary immunodeficiency

One often hears today of the term 'the *compromised host*'. Such patients are generally found in renal, leukaemic, oncological, or intensive care units and are considered 'compromised' because their 'immune defences are low', either due to serious illness, or trauma, or intentional depression of the immune response by drugs during the course of management of a serious disease process.

Many less seriously ill hospitalized patients are also immunologically 'compromised' in a minor way by some of the procedures that are used in their day-to-day management.

Since the last edition of this book early fears that AIDS would emerge as a significant and extremely worrying secondary immune deficiency have been substantiated. This condition has been dealt with in a separate section.

SOME EXAMPLES OF PROCEDURES AND CONDITIONS WHICH 'COMPROMISE' A PATIENT

SKIN DISORDERS:
> e.g. burns
> severe eczema

MALNUTRITION OR MALABSORPTION:
> If protein malabsorption or malnutrition is severe, insufficient immunoglobulin may be synthesized.

LOSS OF PROTEIN:
> Some gut conditions are associated with a protein-losing enteropathy, and in some renal conditions large amounts of protein are lost in the urine. These conditions are often associated with low circulating levels of immunoglobulin.

URINARY CATHETERIZATION:
> Prolonged catheterization provides a focus of infection in the bladder leading to possible pyelonephritis.

INTRAVENOUS CANNULATION:
> This may provide a focus of infection in the circulation, leading to possible septicaemia.

ARTIFICIAL PROSTHESES:
> Artificial valves, hip and other prostheses are avascular foreign bodies. Since the cells of the immune system do not have free access to these areas they can be regarded as 'local' sites of immunodeficiency. Low-grade infection with unusual organisms is not uncommon at such sites.

ANTIBIOTIC THERAPY:
> One of our natural defence mechanisms is the presence of a mixed normal flora of microorganisms. Antibiotic therapy can easily disrupt this healthy symbiotic relationship, leading to colonization by organisms which may eventually gain the upper hand and lead to serious and sometimes unmanageable infection in the host.

TUMOURS:
> Many patients with malignant disease have impairment of one or more branches of the immune system. This may be directly due to the tumour itself or be the result of immunosuppressive agents or radiotherapy used in treatment.

VIRAL INFECTIONS:
> For decades many nurses involved in caring for patients with infection have noticed that a child who is normally Mantoux-positive is likely to become Mantoux-negative during the course of infection with measles virus. This indicates temporary depression of the cell-mediated response during the course of a viral infection. Phagocytic function can also be depressed during the course of some viral infections. The acquired immune deficiency syndrome (AIDS) is an extreme example of the detrimental effect a viral infection can have on the immune system.

IMMUNOSUPPRESSIVE DRUGS:
> The effects of agents such as steroids and azathioprine on the immune system are obviously profound and will be discussed in more detail later.

The neutropenic patient

Infection in the 'compromised host' — a difficult diagnosis

'Normal' patient
with infection

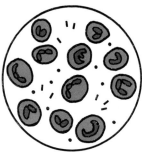

Pus cells and organisms

Neutropenic patient
with infection

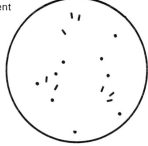

Organisms but no pus cells
No microscopic evidence of infection

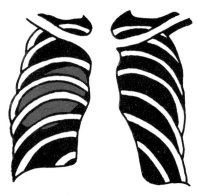

CXR — consolidation

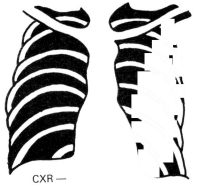

CXR —
**No gross abnormality
but patient has severe pneumonia**

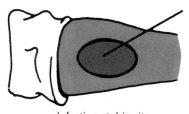

Infection at drip site
— swollen, red, tender.

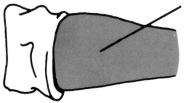

Infection at drip site
No apparent inflammatory response

The neutropenic patient

Phagocytic defects can be classified into two groups:

A. Low numbers of cells (*neutropenia*).
B. Normal numbers of cells but with defective function.

By far the commonest phagocytic deficiency is *neutropenia secondary to immunosuppressive therapy*. During the course of such therapy (e.g. in acute leukaemia) it is necessary, if possible, to kill all the malignant cells present in the host. Unfortunately, during the course of treatment normal cells are also damaged. The white blood count for a time during therapy can fall to almost zero and patients frequently suffer from serious and severe infections. Such a neutropenic patient is an extreme example of a *'compromised host'* and requires a great deal of medical and nursing care to see him through this critical period. Sadly, nevertheless, it is not uncommon for immunosuppressive therapy to be successful in treating the patient's leukaemia and yet death occurs from overwhelming infection. A similar situation exists in patients undergoing bone marrow transplantation.

The diagnosis of infection in the 'compromised host'

All medical students learn the five signs: '*calor*'—heat, '*rubror*'—redness, '*dolor*'—pain, '*tumor*'—swelling, and loss of function of the affected part, which describe the classical signs and symptoms of inflammation. However, in the neutropenic patient these 'rules' of our early teachings are broken, because without neutrophils the patient becomes unable to mount an adequate inflammatory response. Shown opposite are some of the dilemmas facing the physician in the diagnosis of infection in these patients.

Organisms responsible for infection in the 'compromised host'

Some organisms are well known to be responsible for infective disease. *Staphyloccus aureus*, for example, commonly causes boils and carbuncles and, less frequently, pneumonia and septicaemia. *Streptococcus pyogenes* causes cellulitis, erysipelas and throat infections, and the pneumococcus is responsible for lobar pneumonia. These organisms can cause serious and severe infection in neutropenic patients, but more commonly such patients are infected by organisms that generally are considered to be relatively harmless because they are part of the 'normal flora'. Inside the gastrointestinal tract, for example, reside a host of many types of bacteria such as *Escherichia coli*, proteus, bacteroides, some types of streptococci and *Clostridium welchii*. Such a mixed normal flora is in a way protective since it prevents more pathogenic organisms becoming established. In a patient receiving immunosuppressive therapy, however, some problems arise.

Alterations of the normal flora

Potent immunosuppressive drugs can be toxic to resident bacteria and can alter the 'balance' of mixed flora, allowing a preponderance of a particular type of organism. Antibiotic therapy can have a similar effect. An organism thus established is more liable to cause infection.

Ulceration of the mucous membranes

The cells lining the mucous membranes are themselves frequently damaged by immunosuppressive therapy and this leads to ulceration. The organisms within the gastrointestinal and respiratory tracts, therefore, readily gain access to the circulation through the damaged mucous membrane and septicaemia may result.

Bacteriological screens

Since infection in the neutropenic patient is difficult to diagnose, it is sometimes helpful to do frequent screens of bacteriological specimens from such patients in order to detect the presence of highly pathogenic organisms so that they can be eradicated before infection is established, and to identify the antibiotic sensitivities of the patient's normal flora so that a 'best guess' combination of antibiotics can be used immediately if the patient becomes ill.

Unfortunately, if infection is present, any delay in giving antibiotic therapy may be rapidly fatal, and thus treatment often has to be given before the cause of infection is established.

Often, the appearance of pus in an infected neutropenic patient with leukaemia is a good sign since it means that his white count is recovering and his leukaemia is going into remission.

Protective isolation

Although most incidents of infection in a neutropenic patient are the result of invasion from his own organisms, it is important to prevent the access of new organisms from the environment. Hence, these patients should be nursed in a single room, or in a laminar flow bed, during the time that the granulocyte count has fallen to its lowest level. Great care should be taken with oral hygiene, intravenous drip sites, and dressings during this time.

Bacteriological screening of the immunosuppressed patient

On admission–prior to immunosuppression	Thereafter–during immunosuppression

• Nasal swabs
• Mouth swabs
• Throat swab
• Sputum (if available)
• Urine
• Stool
• Skin – Axillae: Umbilicus: Groins: Skin lesions
  – Look for *Staphylococcus aureus*, pseudomonas, Group A streptococcus, pneumococcus, Fungi
  – Note the antibiotic sensitivity pattern of the normal flora
	• Nasal swabs
	• Mouth swab
	• Throat swab
	• Sputum (if available)
	• Urine
	• Stool
	• Skin – Restrict to skin lesions, drip sites
	  Full screen on previous carriers of *Staphylococcus aureus*

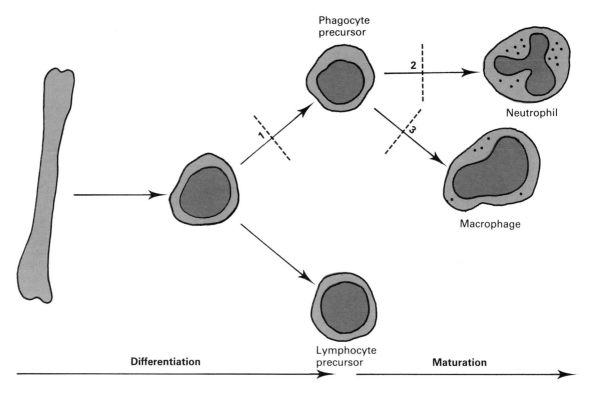

Phagocyte precursor

Neutrophil

Macrophage

Lymphocyte precursor

Differentiation

Maturation

Primary immunodeficiency

In 1952 Bruton described the first serious primary immunodeficiency. Since then, various syndromes have been recognized. These syndromes are sometimes referred to as 'experiments of nature' since they have taught immunologists a great deal about the normal immune response. The primary immune deficiencies can be described under four headings:

1. *Deficiencies of non-specific immunity.*
2. *Deficiencies of humoral immunity.*
3. *Deficiencies of cell-mediated immunity.*
4. *Combined deficiencies.*

Deficiencies of non-specific immunity

In spite of the complexity of the immune system in mammals, the mainstay of their body defences is still largely dependent on surface barriers and phagocytic mechanisms. It is not surprising, therefore, that defects in these systems are associated with severe infections.

It should be noted also that, in many situations, chemotaxis and phagocytosis by neutrophils is dependent on the production of chemotactic factors liberated during the course of complement activation. Complement defects may therefore manifest as neutrophil function defects.

Phagocytic defects

Phagocytic defects may be classified into two groups:

1. *Low* numbers of cells—*neutropenia*
2. *Normal* numbers of cells but with *defective function*

Neutropenias—The normal neutrophil count in blood is 2500–7500 per mm^3. A drop in the count from these levels becomes dangerous when the value falls to less than 500 per mm^3. *Secondary neutropenia* caused by drugs, radiation therapy, or associated with other conditions such as autoimmune disease, is much commoner than the *congenital primary neutropenias* which are fortunately very rare. An example of a primary disorder is *cyclic neutropenia*, a condition in which the neutrophil count falls in a cyclical manner and then recovers only to fall again. Antibody synthesis and cell-mediated responses are functionally intact in most, since the abnormality in maturation of the neutrophils probably occurs at stage 2 in the diagram above.

Functional defects—These may be classified into:

1. *Defective chemotaxis*
2. *Defective ingestion and digestion*
3. *Defective opsonization*

Normal inflammatory response

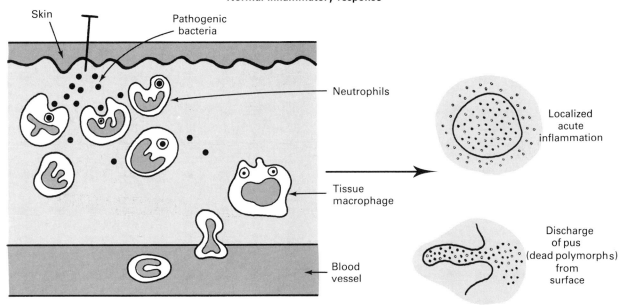

The inflammatory response associated with neutrophil defects

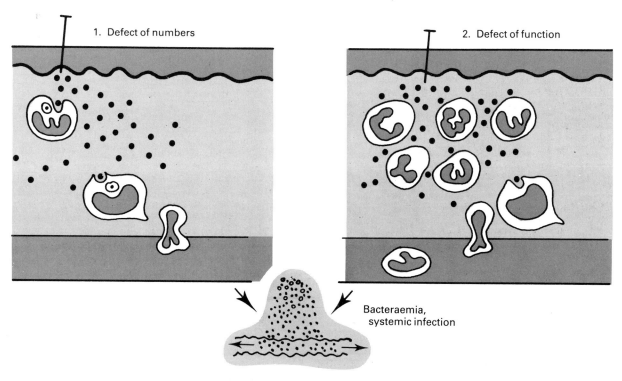

Defective chemotaxis—The localization of phagocytes in an inflammatory site depends on the generation of chemotactic mediators and a directional response by cells. These processes fail when the polymorphs themselves are abnormal, where there is a complement system defect, or where there are serum inhibitors of chemotaxis.

Defective ingestion and digestion—There are a number of rare paediatric syndromes due to defective intracellular killing by macrophages and neutrophils. These children have a history of repeated bacterial infections, e.g. chronic lymph node enlargement with sinus formation, respiratory infections, and skin infections. The abnormality in maturation of the phagocytes occurs at stage 1 of the diagram.

Defective opsonization—Rarely, a defect can occur in the complement system or in antibody synthesis which leads to a defect in the coating of a microorganism by antibody or products of the complement system. This leads to defective phagocytosis since the phagocyte can recognize 'coated' or 'opsonized' microorganisms more easily.

Complement deficiencies

Some rare conditions exist where certain components of the complement system are absent. Not only do these patients suffer from an increased incidence of infection as described above but there also appears to be a higher incidence of autoimmune disease than in the normal population.

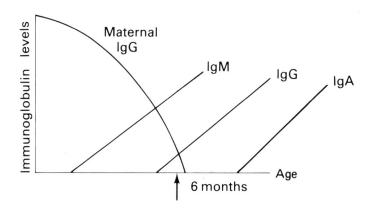

Normal physiological immunoglobulin deficiency in a baby

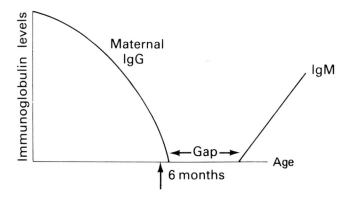

Transient hypogammaglobulinaemia of infancy

Deficiencies of humoral immunity

Transient hypogammaglobulinaemia of infancy

There are some common infectious diseases (e.g. measles) that one very seldom sees in this country in children before the age of six months. This is because maternal IgG has crossed the placenta during foetal life, and since most women have antibody to measles virus this offers 'passive' protection to the newborn.

By the age of six months maternal IgG reaches a fairly low level, but most infants have started to produce their own immunoglobulin by this time (IgM first, followed later by IgG and then IgA). Since the child's own immune system has not by this time experienced challenge by most of the common infectious agents, there is a tendency to suffer clinical infection during childhood until most common antigens have been met, and immunological 'memory' is built up.

Very occasionally in some infants there is a delay in onset of immunoglobulin synthesis, so that there may be a temporary period of agammaglobulinaemia until the age of eighteen months or so. During this time they may well suffer from recurrent bacterial infections and these may be severe enough or frequent enough to warrant treatment with injections of gammaglobulin.

Bruton's hypogammaglobulinaemia

This genetically determined condition may be difficult to distinguish from transient hypogammaglobulinaemia of infancy during early years. During the first six months of life, these children are of course protected to some extent by maternal IgG. After six months, bacterial infection becomes a problem because all classes of immunoglobulin are absent or extremely low. This is a permanent state of affairs which does not improve as the child matures. The condition appears to affect only the humoral branch of the immune system—T cell function and non-specific immunity appear to be normal.

Treatment involves the avoidance of infection, appropriate antibiotic therapy where indicated, and gammaglobulin injections every 3–4 weeks, and perhaps also plasma infusions. With proper management, these patients can survive well into adulthood.

Common variable hypogammaglobulinaemia

This condition, also associated with low levels of all classes of immunoglobulin, does not present until young adult life. There is generally no history of recurrent infection in childhood, suggesting that immunoglobulin levels are normal initially. There is some evidence to suggest that the deficiency lies in the regulation of antibody synthesis by B cells, since these cells are present in normal numbers in this condition.

Treatment is identical to that of Bruton's hypogammaglobulinaemia. If managed well, these patients have a good prognosis.

Selective IgA deficiency

This is the most common primary immunodeficiency syndrome, in which IgA is absent but IgG and IgM are present in normal amounts. Patients may live a completely normal life and be unaware that they have a problem. Alternatively, they may suffer from respiratory infections or diarrhoeal disease, or occasionally present with autoimmune disease or tumours.

Treatment of these patients is supportive, with avoidance of infection, treatment of respiratory infections with antibiotics, and management of diarrhoea. Unlike the other B cell deficiencies, gammaglobulin injections should not be given, because the IgA contained in these preparations may be recognized as 'foreign' and a patient's IgG antibodies produced against it. This may result in a hypersensitivity reaction. For the same reasons blood transfusions are not without risk in these patients.

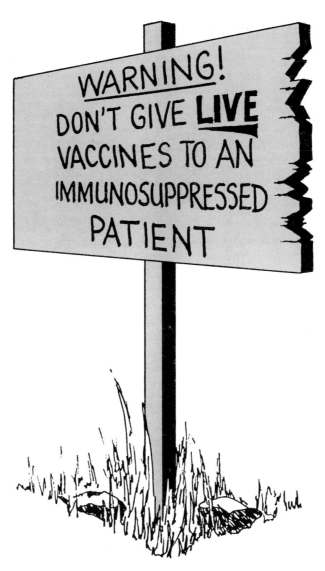

Deficiencies of cell–mediated immunity

Di George's syndrome

This condition is the result of a developmental abnormality of the third and fourth pharyngeal pouches. This results in absence of the thymus and is also associated with an abnormality in parathyroid development. These infants generally present in the neonatal period with *hypocalcaemic tetany*. The child generally goes on to develop recurrent viral, fungal, or protozoal infections and without early diagnosis and treatment the outlook is bleak.

The T cell deficiency can be reversed by implanting *foetal thymic tissue*, but experience in the long-term management of these patients into adulthood is as yet limited.

At this point it is worth emphasizing that immunodeficient patients can suffer severe and sometimes fatal infections from organisms that are not usually considered to be pathogenic. For this reason 'live' vaccines should never be given to an immuno-suppressed patient since even attenuated organisms can cause infection.

Summary of primary deficiencies of the immune response

A
> **Deficiencies of non-specific immunity**
>
> Phagocytic defects
> (1) Neutropenia
> (2) Defective function — chemotaxis, ingestion
> and killing, opsonization
> Complement deficiencies

B
> **Deficiencies of humoral immunity**
>
> Transient hypogammaglobulinaemia of infancy
> Bruton's hypogammaglobulinaemia
> Common variable hypogammaglobulinaemia
> Selective IgA deficiency

C
> **Deficiencies of cell-mediated immunity**
>
> Di George's syndrome

D
> **Combined deficiencies**
>
> Severe combined immune deficiency

Combined deficiencies

Swiss–type agammaglobulinaemia (severe combined immunodeficiency)

This is the most severe type of immunodeficiency and generally leads to death in early childhood. Both humoral and cell-mediated limbs of the immune response are involved and these children suffer from infections with all types of microorganisms. This disease may be a result of a defect in the bone marrow stem cell. In some patients there also seems to be an absence of the enzyme *adenosine deaminase*.

Bacterial infection should be treated with antibiotics, but eventually these children succumb to infections with organisms not amenable to such therapy. Bone marrow transplantation, thymic transplant and foetal liver transplant, along with immunoglobulin therapy have been attempted; however, the outlook for these children remains poor, but advances in knowledge and techniques may well improve the prognosis substantially during the next decade.

Why does autoimmune disease occur?

Exposure of 'new' antigens

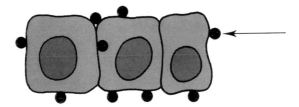

Normal tissue antigens regarded as 'self' and no immune response is mounted

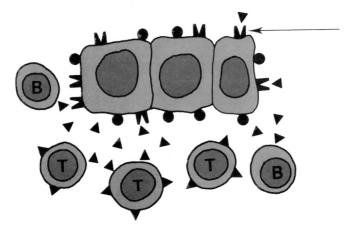

Damaged or infected tissue may sometimes reveal 'new' antigens which the individual does not regard as 'self'. A humoral and cell-mediated response is mounted

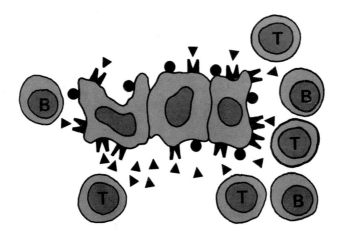

Tissue destruction occurs. This may result in a 'vicious circle' with exposure of more new antigens

14. Autoimmune disease

Autoimmunity

In the *normal, healthy state, self antigens* are clearly distinguished from *foreign antigens* and immunological damage against an individual's own tissues does not occur. It is not known whether the immune response to self antigens is normally completely absent or whether it is present but greatly diminished.

In the *autoimmune state* the immune response of an individual is directed against his body's own constituents. This may involve B cells, or T cells, or both limbs of the response. An *autoimmune response*, however, does not necessarily imply that *autoimmune disease* is present. For example, a patient suffering from *pernicious anaemia* almost invariably has circulating autoantibodies directed specifically against his own gastric tissue, but apparently healthy individuals with no symptoms or signs of pernicious anaemia can also have circulating gastric antibodies.

Why does autoimmune disease occur?

Some years ago, autoimmune disease was considered to be a 'byproduct' of an overactive immune system. It came as a surprise, therefore, to find that there was an association between autoimmune disease and immunodeficiency states. In these patients there is an increased immunological response to self antigens in the face of a deficient response to some or all foreign antigens. The mechanisms leading to autoimmunity in these patients are not fully understood, but it is now clear that the concept of overactivity of the immune system was a simplistic one. Several theories are discussed below. They may be proven or disproven in the near future. However, it is not unlikely that several mechanisms may be responsible.

Probably autoimmune disease can occur by two main mechanisms:

1. *Alteration in the host tissue*
2. *Alteration in the immune response*

Alteration in host tissue

Antigenic alteration

Sometimes the antigenic configuration of host tissues can undergo a change. Damage to a cell by trauma or infection of a cell by, for example, a virus, may uncover hidden antigenic determinants or add completely new antigenic determinants. The host's immune system will then recognize the altered tissues as 'foreign' and mount an immune response against them.

Exposure of sequestered antigens

Some normal tissues are 'hidden' or 'sequestered' from the immune system, i.e. the immune system has at no time met these antigens and therefore is not programmed to regard them as 'self'. If as a result of injury these tissues become exposed to the immune system, a damaging reaction results. *Lens protein*, for example, is a sequestered antigen. If this protein is released into the circulation (e.g. during surgery), inflammatory changes affecting the lens protein of the other eye may result, leading to the condition of *uveitis*.

Upset in suppressor–helper control mechanisms

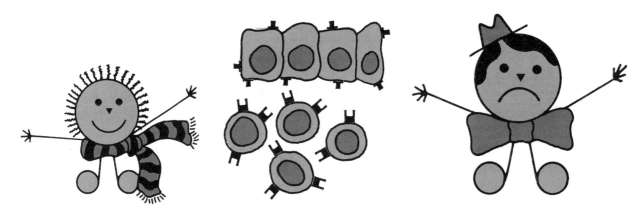

Suppressor and helper controlling mechanisms may be important in autoimmune disease

Normal state — predominance of suppressor activity

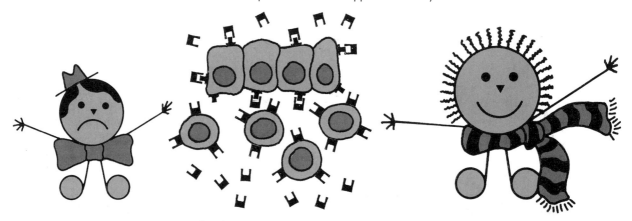

Autoimmune state — loss of suppressor activity
or excess of helper activity

Alteration in the immune response

Cross-reactivity

Sometimes an immune reaction may be mounted against a microorganism in which some antigenic determinants are similar to some of the host's own tissues. Antibody made may then be weakly *cross-reactive* against self and autoimmune disease may result.

Suppressor–helper T cell imbalance

If one accepts the simplified concept that both humoral and cell-mediated responses are increased by helper T cell function and decreased by suppressor T cell function, then it is possible that quantitative or qualitative deficiencies in these cells could have serious consequences on the immune response. It is possible, for example, if suppressor T cells are functioning inadequately, that tolerance to one's own tissues can be lost and autoimmune disease result (see p. 35).

A summary of some of the conditions normally regarded as autoimmune follows. Other common conditions may well, in the fullness of time, be shown to have an autoimmune basis.

Examples of some autoimmune diseases

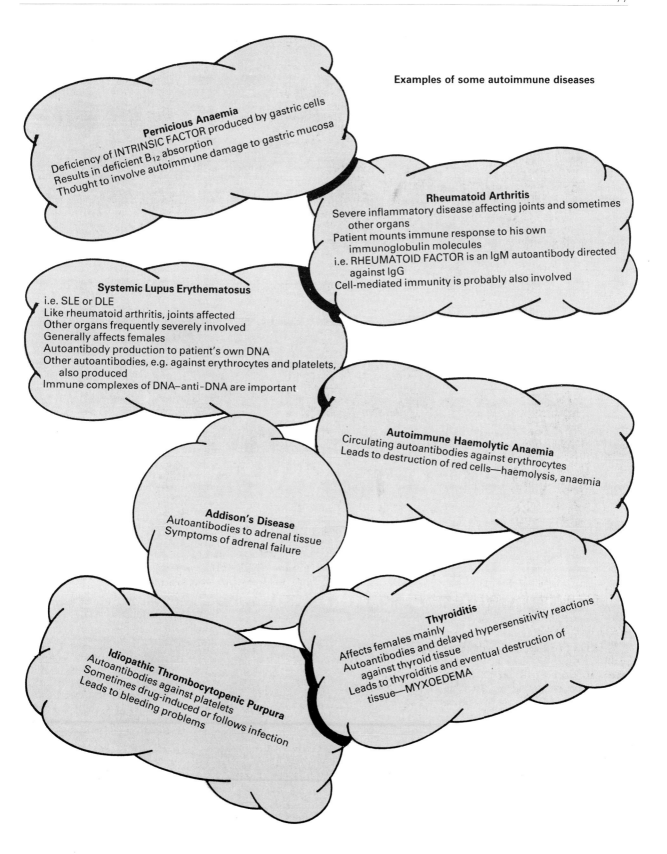

Pernicious Anaemia
Deficiency of INTRINSIC FACTOR produced by gastric cells
Results in deficient B$_{12}$ absorption
Thought to involve autoimmune damage to gastric mucosa

Rheumatoid Arthritis
Severe inflammatory disease affecting joints and sometimes other organs
Patient mounts immune response to his own immunoglobulin molecules
i.e. RHEUMATOID FACTOR is an IgM autoantibody directed against IgG
Cell-mediated immunity is probably also involved

Systemic Lupus Erythematosus
i.e. SLE or DLE
Like rheumatoid arthritis, joints affected
Other organs frequently severely involved
Generally affects females
Autoantibody production to patient's own DNA
Other autoantibodies, e.g. against erythrocytes and platelets, also produced
Immune complexes of DNA–anti-DNA are important

Autoimmune Haemolytic Anaemia
Circulating autoantibodies against erythrocytes
Leads to destruction of red cells—haemolysis, anaemia

Addison's Disease
Autoantibodies to adrenal tissue
Symptoms of adrenal failure

Idiopathic Thrombocytopenic Purpura
Autoantibodies against platelets
Sometimes drug-induced or follows infection
Leads to bleeding problems

Thyroiditis
Affects females mainly
Autoantibodies and delayed hypersensitivity reactions against thyroid tissue
Leads to thyroiditis and eventual destruction of tissue—MYXOEDEMA

Polyclonal versus monoclonal gammopathy

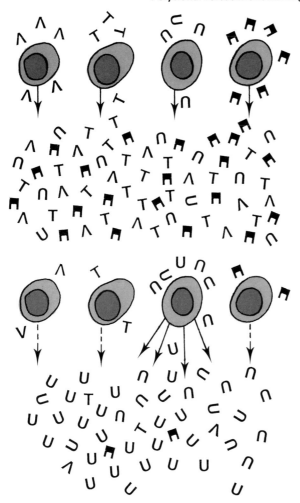

Polyclonal gammopathy

Increased numbers of several
different antibody molecules

Antibody normal and
functional

Monoclonal gammopathy

Increased numbers of one type
of antibody molecule

This monoclonal antibody is
often of bizarre structure
and has no protective function

Normal antibody synthesis
from other clones of plasma
cells is depressed

15. The monoclonal gammopathies

Sometimes due to prolonged antigenic stimulation, one or more classes of immunoglobulin can reach levels that are much higher than normal. This is due to the production of antibodies against the whole range of antigenic determinants present on the stimulating antigen. Such a diverse increase in immunoglobulin is known as a *polyclonal gammopathy*.

On the other hand, a single plasma cell may divide to form a 'clone' of cells, all capable of producing a single identical type of immunoglobulin molecule. Very often these plasma cells are malignant and the patient presents clinically with symptoms and signs of a bony tumour. The immunoglobulin molecules produced are often bizarre, fragmented, and function-

less. Normal immunoglobulins are depressed and so there is a paradoxical picture of immunological deficiency in spite of very high immunoglobulin levels.

Multiple myeloma

The plasma cells in multiple myeloma are capable of producing one class of immunoglobulin only: either IgG, IgA, IgD, or IgE (IgG is the commonest type, IgE the rarest). If the immunoglobulin produced is fragmented, free light chains may be produced. These are small enough to pass into the urine as *Bence-Jones protein.* (Bence-Jones proteinuria was described long before myeloma was understood. When the urine is heated to 60 °C, Bence-Jones protein precipitates. On heating further, the protein redissolves.)

Waldenstrom's macroglobulinaemia

This is the name given to an IgM-secreting 'myeloma'. It is regarded as a separate entity since the clinical symptoms are different from myeloma.

Since IgM is a large molecule, many of the symptoms are due to the hyperviscosity created by the large amounts of circulating IgM.

Light chain disease and heavy chain disease

Sometimes only light chains are produced by malignant plasma cells, and sometimes only heavy chains.

Transplantation terminology

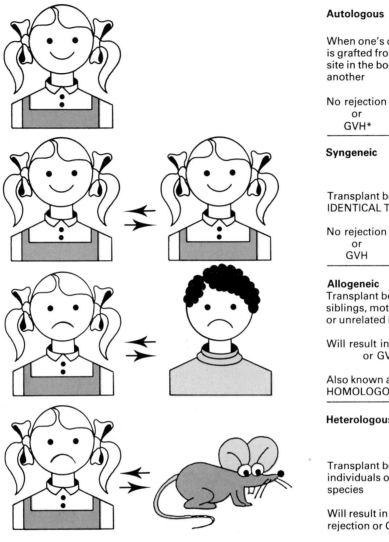

Autologous

When one's own tissue
is grafted from one
site in the body to
another

No rejection
or
GVH*

Syngeneic

Transplant between
IDENTICAL TWINS

No rejection
or
GVH

Allogeneic
Transplant between
siblings, mother and child,
or unrelated individuals

Will result in rejection
or GVH

Also known as a
HOMOLOGOUS GRAFT

Heterologous or xenogeneic

Transplant between
individuals of different
species

Will result in
rejection or GVH

* GVH = Graft versus host disease

16. Transplantation immunology

Some terminology

When a blood transfusion is given, a great deal of immunological damage can result unless the blood is *cross-matched*, i.e. the red blood cells of the donor must be *compatible* with those of the recipient. For example, a patient who is A positive would be expected to have a *transfusion reaction* if given blood from a B positive donor. In the same way, when a tissue is transplanted, the cells of the donor and recipient must be compatible. The term *'tissue typing'* in *transplantation* is equivalent to *'cross-matching'* in *blood transfusion*, and the term *'rejection'* is equivalent to the term *'transfusion reaction'*.

An individual's tissue cells and lymphocytes have certain antigens on their membranes. Lymphocytes in particular have large amounts of these surface antigens and so they have been given the name *human lymphocyte antigens* (commonly abbreviated to HLA). The types of HLA antigens possessed by each individual are genetically determined. In man, the genes known as the *major histocompatibility genes* responsible for an individual's HLA type reside on the *sixth chromosome*. (These HLA genes are incidentally situated very close to the genes that decide an individual's ability to mount good or poor responses to antigens. These are known as *immune response* or Ir genes.)

The only situation in the human where a transplant can be performed without the problem of rejection is where normal healthy tissue is transplanted from one identical twin to another. This is because they are genetically totally compatible.

In summary, for a transplant to be successful, both *blood group antigens* and *tissue antigens* must be compatible.

Privileged grafts

Some tissues are not exposed to lymphocytes, therefore an immune response against grafts to these areas does not result. This is true of *corneal grafts*, and when this is performed the rules of tissue histocompatibility can be ignored.

Immunological reactions associated with transplantation

Rejection

Three types of rejection have been recognized and in each case different immunological mechanisms are involved.

Immunological reactions associated with transplantation

A. Rejection

Hyperacute rejection
occurs when an individual has antibody prior to transplantation of donor tissue

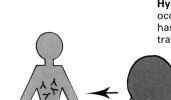

Acute rejection
occurs 2–4 weeks following transplantation. Results from a cell-mediated reaction

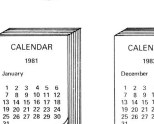

Chronic rejection
occurs months or years after transplantation.
Results from weak immune response to a slightly incompatible graft

B. Graft versus host disease

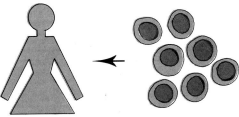

Results when immunologically competent cells are transplanted

Immunodeficient recipient   Immunocompetent graft

1. *Hyperacute rejection*. If an individual already possesses antibodies to the transplant, this type of rejection results. These antibodies could have been made on a previous occasion as a result of numerous blood transfusions, or numerous pregnancies (the foetus is foreign to the mother, i.e. HLA incompatible), or even from a previous transplant. In this type of rejection, the graft never 'takes'—there is widespread vascular occlusion around the grafted organ and the graft is very quickly destroyed.

   Obviously a search for such antibodies in the patient's serum prior to transplant is an important part of the work of a tissue-typing laboratory.

2. *Acute rejection*. This reaction is seen 2–4 weeks after transplantation and is the result of a cell-mediated response involving T lymphocytes.

3. *Chronic rejection*. Although one tries to graft from an ABO and HLA compatible donor, generally one must settle for a graft where there are minor differences (not necessarily identified in the laboratory) between donor and recipient. Immunosuppressive therapy following transplantation may prevent this becoming a problem. However, months or years following a renal transplant there may be a gradual loss of kidney function due to a slow rejection process.

Graft versus host disease

If the transplanted tissue consists of immunologically active cells such as *bone marrow cells*, then the graft itself may mount an immune response against the host, i.e. instead of the host rejecting the transplant, the transplant rejects the host! It is extremely important, therefore, that bone marrow transplants are compatible. During graft versus host disease, the graft recipient experiences numerous symptoms such as skin rashes, loss of weight and diarrhoea. If the symptoms are not recognized, and the graft removed, the patient may die.

The present status of organ transplantation

Since the early 1960s attempts have been made with varying degrees of success to transplant kidneys, heart, liver, lungs, pancreas and bone marrow. Of these only kidney and bone marrow transplantation are as yet accepted without reservation as successful and the treatment of choice in certain circumstances.

Much of the success of kidney transplantation is due to the fact that transplantation is possible from a well-matched living donor. The success rate with cadaveric donors is not so high, although continuing improvements in tissue matching and preservation of renal tissue after death may alter this.

Unlike other organ transplantations, bone marrow transplantation is an extremely easy procedure; however, graft versus host disease and opportunistic infections remain a major problem. It is now an accepted management of certain types of leukaemia and is also used in the treatment of aplastic anaemia and in the very severe but rare form of congenital immune deficiency known as SCID (severe combined immune deficiency).

Cyclosporin A is an immunosuppressive agent that has in recent years led to an improvement in rejection rate following all types of transplantation. This does not create the same severity of side effects seen with some other agents.

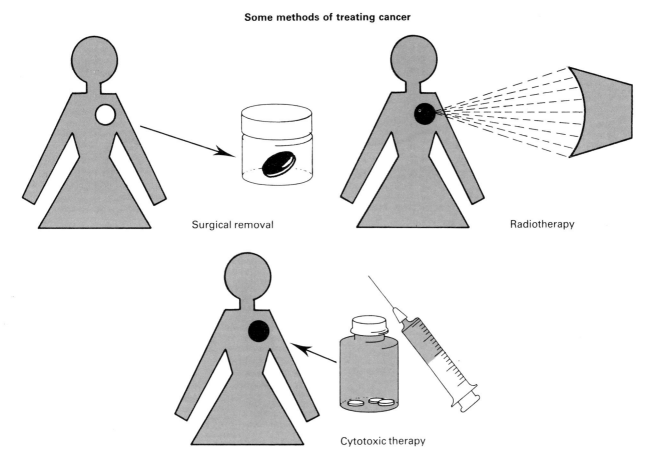

Some methods of treating cancer

Surgical removal

Radiotherapy

Cytotoxic therapy

17. Tumour immunology

What is cancer?

When a normal cell grows it obeys a set of rules which instruct it to *differentiate* into a certain type of tissue and to *proliferate* until it reaches a certain size. The regulatory mechanisms necessary to ensure that cells conform to these rules are poorly understood, but it is clear that when they break down a state of chaos that we call cancer supervenes.

Malignant cells generally are poorly differentiated, grow rapidly and spread as *metastases* throughout the body with little regard for the normal healthy tissues that they replace. Such widespread cancer is probably the result of malignant change in one single cell.

In these circumstances we try to help the patient by using some fairly crude methods. We surgically remove the tumour, irradiate it, or try to destroy it by giving cytotoxic drugs—drugs which will also to a greater or lesser extent have an action on normal tissues, especially rapidly reproducing cells like those of bone marrow.

Sometimes we try to stimulate the patient's own defences so that he can destroy his tumour. In doing this, we are at present largely groping in the dark since we do not yet fully understand the natural mechanisms involved in tumour prevention.

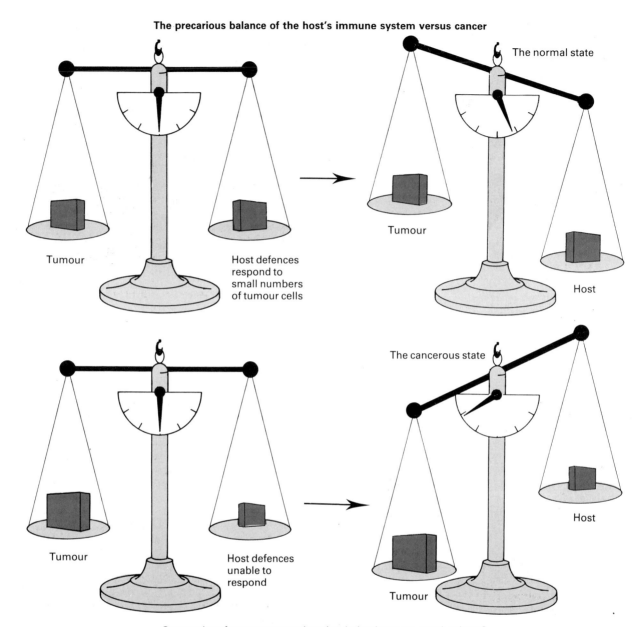

The precarious balance of the host's immune system versus cancer

Tumour

Host defences respond to small numbers of tumour cells

The normal state

Tumour

Host

Tumour

Host defences unable to respond

The cancerous state

Host

Tumour

Can we therefore treat cancer by stimulating immune mechanisms?

Cancer—a precarious balance!

It is very likely that malignant transformation of single cells is not an uncommon event. Probably all of us, many times during our lifetime, cope with these potential 'cancers' by eradicating them as soon as they develop. The part our immune system plays in this process is a matter of some controversy. Some immunologists take the view that immunity has a minor role to play in tumour prevention, while others feel that this is one of its main functions. At the moment the evidence shows that immunology does have an important but very unpredictable role to play—indeed, sometimes the immune system behaves in such a way that it appears to help rather than to hinder growth.

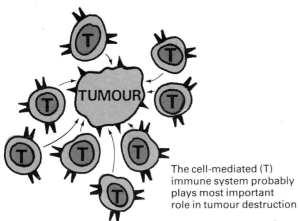

Tumour-specific antibody produced by B cells prevents more efficiently destructive T cells from gaining access

The cell-mediated (T) immune system probably plays most important role in tumour destruction

Antibody-producing (B) cells play a minor role

i.e. Tumour destruction

i.e. Blocking antibody → enhancement of tumour growth

Tumours as antigens

If the specific immune system is to function in a protective way against tumour formation, then the tumour itself must be antigenic to the host, i.e. unlike the tissue of origin it must be regarded as foreign.

There is evidence that when a cell becomes malignant new surface antigens appear which are recognized by the host as non-self, and an immune response involving both humoral and cell-mediated immunity is initiated. Sometimes these antigens are similar to those found on embryonic tissue, emphasizing the primitive nature of some tumours. Examples of such de-differentiated tumour antigens are *alphafoetoprotein* associated with *hepatomas* and *carcinoembryonic antigen* associated with *carcinoma of the colon*. It is worth noting that about 15% of heavy smokers also have raised serum levels of this antigen, suggesting that de-differentiation has occurred in the absence of frank tumour formation.

It is interesting that a tumour caused by an *oncogenic virus* has the same surface antigens as tumours in other individuals caused by the same virus. On the other hand, tumours induced by *chemical carcinogens* produce antigenic changes that are unique for each individual tumour.

The host's immune response to tumours—sometimes protective, sometimes harmful

Probably, once a tumour reaches a certain size, the immune system, even if working with maximum efficiency, will be quite unable to cope, and the tumour will grow relentlessly. It is likely, therefore,

that the most important role of the immune system is at a very early stage of tumour formation, or in the 'mopping up' of residual cancer cells after surgery and irradiation.

There has over the years been some controversy about the role of the *cell-mediated system* in tumour protection. Current opinion suggests it may have an important role to play in the earliest stages of tumour formation. CMI however, is only part of the anti-tumour orchestra; there is no doubt that macrophages, complement, NK cells and to a lesser extent antibody also play a role.

It is likely that an adequate immune response results only if the antigenic structure of the tumour is not too similar to the antigenic structure of the tissue from which it was derived. If the tumour is antigenically only slightly different from the host tissues, a weak immune response or even tolerance may result.

Sometimes the body can produce antibody against a developing tumour, but instead of inhibiting growth the antibody coats the tumour cells protecting them from the effects of cell-mediated immune response. Hence there is a tendency to feel that humoral immune responses to tumours are harmful, whereas cell-mediated responses are protective. This, however, is probably an oversimplification of the situation.

There is increasing evidence that non-specific immune mechanisms in the form of macrophages and natural killer cells (NK cells) have an important role to play. These mechanisms come into action quicker than specific immune responses.

It is of interest that both cell-mediated immunity and natural killer cell activity are considerably lower at the extremes of life, correlating well with the times when individuals are much more prone to develop malignancies.

Immunotherapy—exciting future possibilities for the treatment of cancer

Surgical removal of tumours, irradiation and conventional cytotoxic therapy are likely to be with us for a long time to come; however, there is growing evidence that more sophisticated highly selective therapy will become available in the near future.

Monoclonal antibodies can now be made in the laboratory against certain types of tumour (see p. 176). They have two important potential uses: A. *diagnostically* and B. *therapeutically*.

A. The diagnostic use of monoclonal antibodies

One important problem has always been to locate tumour metastases. A monoclonal antibody in which the Fab ends of the molecule have exquisite specificity for the tumour antigens in question can be linked to a radioactive substance. The 'labelled' antibody can then be injected intravenously. It then 'seeks out' any deposits of tumour cells throughout the body and these can be detected using radiological techniques.

Another problem has been to detect at a very early stage when a tumour is reappearing after curative therapy has been attempted. Certain tumours secrete their primitive embryonic structures into the surrounding environment (e.g. alphafoetoprotein as already described). This reaches the blood stream. Tiny amounts of this and similar substances can now be detected in the laboratory from a patient's blood sample using monoclonal antibodies to detect the antigen in question. Such an 'early warning' system may be used to indicate when aggressive anti-tumour therapy is indicated.

A diagnostic use of monoclonal antibody

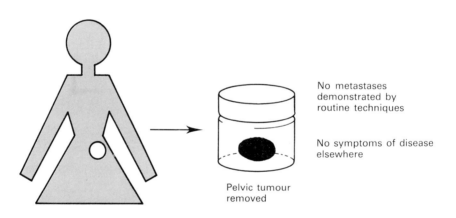

No metastases demonstrated by routine techniques

No symptoms of disease elsewhere

Pelvic tumour removed

But

Is there any undetectable tumour spread?

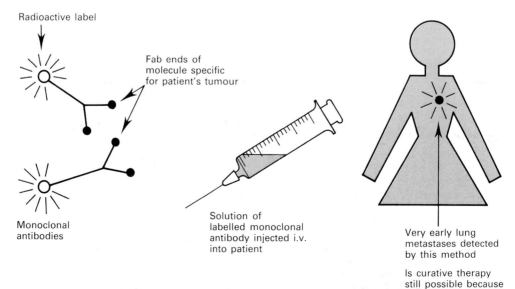

Radioactive label

Fab ends of molecule specific for patient's tumour

Monoclonal antibodies

Solution of labelled monoclonal antibody injected i.v. into patient

Very early lung metastases detected by this method

Is curative therapy still possible because of early detection?

B. The therapeutic use of monoclonal antibodies

The almost unacceptable side-effects of many types of cytotoxic anti-tumour therapy are well known. These effects are due to serious damage to normal body tissues such as in the gastrointestinal tract, bone marrow, hair follicles, etc. What a difference it would make if cytotoxic substances limited their aggression to malignant cells only, leaving the normal cells untouched and able to function normally.

Monoclonal antibodies now mean that such a therapeutic ideal is within the realms of possibility. Theoretically, lethal toxins can be coupled to monoclonal antibodies. Only the tumour cells would be 'sought out' by such a 'magic bullet', resulting in total eradication of the tumour cells without any side-effects to the patient, because all other cells would be unaffected. Such an ideal state has for several reasons not yet been achieved but it remains an area of active research.

A possible future therapeutic use of monoclonal antibody. 'Magic bullet' therapy

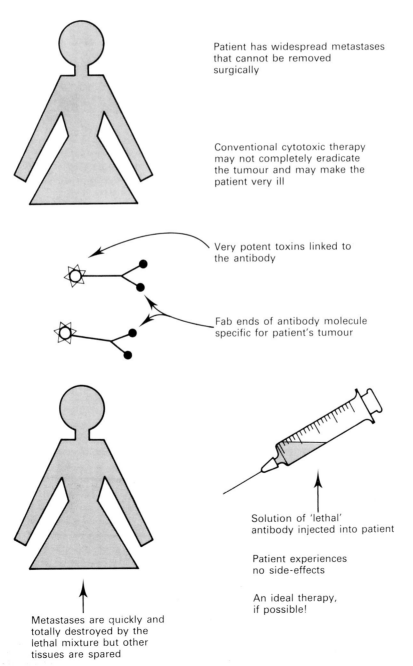

Patient has widespread metastases that cannot be removed surgically

Conventional cytotoxic therapy may not completely eradicate the tumour and may make the patient very ill

Very potent toxins linked to the antibody

Fab ends of antibody molecule specific for patient's tumour

Solution of 'lethal' antibody injected into patient

Patient experiences no side-effects

An ideal therapy, if possible!

Metastases are quickly and totally destroyed by the lethal mixture but other tissues are spared

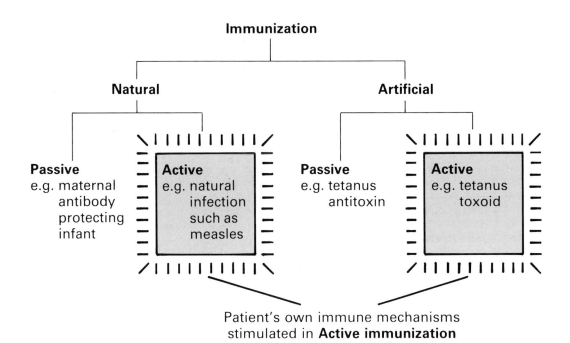

Patient's own immune mechanisms
stimulated in **Active immunization**

18. Immunization

The principles

The aim of immunization is to provoke a *positive* immune response by an individual to various pathogenic microorganisms so as to confer protection against their harmful effects.

Immunization can occur *naturally* or may be induced *artificially*. Both natural and artifically induced immunity may be *passive* or *active*.

Passive immunization

Protection is conferred by giving *preformed* antibody from another immune individual. This protection, however, is short-lived. It is gradually lost as the acquired antibodies are utilized by combination with antigen or catabolized in the normal way.

Examples of passive immunization

Natural mechanisms

Transplacental transfer of antibody—IgG is transferred across the placenta during intrauterine life. At birth, therefore, a baby has substantial amounts of maternal IgG which is protective against many of the common infections that the baby is likely to encounter (e.g. measles, chicken pox, rubella). This passively acquired IgG gradually decays and at about age six months most of this protection is lost. Fortunately, by this time, most infants begin to respond to antigens by producing their own immunoglobulin.

Breast feeding—Human milk and in particular human *colostrum* contains a high concentration of IgA. The breast-fed baby therefore has the advantage of a gastrointestinal tract 'lined' with protective maternal

Passive immunization

A.

> **Human normal immunoglobulin**
> Measles
> Hepatitis A
> Rubella

B.

> **Human specific immunoglobulin**
> Tetanus   Rabies
> Chicken pox   Mumps
> Hepatitis B

C.*

> **Animal specific immunoglobulin**
> Tetanus   Diphtheria
> Gas gangrene   Botulism

* This type of passive immunization is associated with a
considerable risk of anaphylaxis

IgA. This is thought to be one of the reasons why such infants suffer from fewer gastrointestinal infections than bottle-fed babies.

Artificial mechanisms

Gammaglobulin therapy—Passive immunity can be artificially induced by the intramuscular administration of immunoglobulin from the serum of other individuals or animals. This may take the form of *pooled normal human immunoglobulin*. Such a preparation contains adequate antibody levels only to those infections that are very common in the general community. It is therefore, for example, of un-

doubted value in the prevention of *viral hepatitis A or measles*.

When very high antibody levels against a particular organism are required, *human specific immunoglobulin* can be given. For example, if passive protection were required for a patient who had been exposed to *hepatitis B*, human specific immunoglobulin could be prepared from the sera of individuals convalescing from naturally acquired serum hepatitis.

Antitoxin administration—Sometimes serious disease is caused not by a microorganism itself but by one of its harmful products known as a *toxin*. *Diphtheria* and *tetanus* are examples of such diseases. Sometimes it is a matter of urgency to protect a

Passive immunization with human gammaglobulin

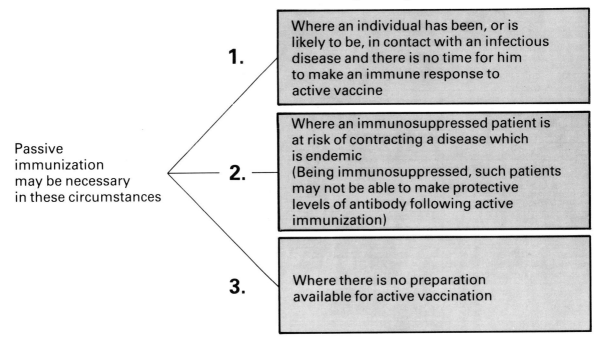

Passive immunization may be necessary in these circumstances

1. Where an individual has been, or is likely to be, in contact with an infectious disease and there is no time for him to make an immune response to active vaccine

2. Where an immunosuppressed patient is at risk of contracting a disease which is endemic (Being immunosuppressed, such patients may not be able to make protective levels of antibody following active immunization)

3. Where there is no preparation available for active vaccination

previously unimmunized individual against these conditions. This is done by the intramuscular administration of *antitoxins*, i.e. serum containing high levels of antibody to the toxin in question. Until fairly recently antitoxins were produced by immunizing horses. The horse serum containing high levels of antibody against the toxin was then injected into the patient at risk. Such a procedure was often followed by a serious hypersensitivity reaction due to the patient recognizing horse serum as 'foreign'. More recently, human antiserum has become available for many conditions and this, although more expensive, should be used whenever possible.

Passive versus active immunization

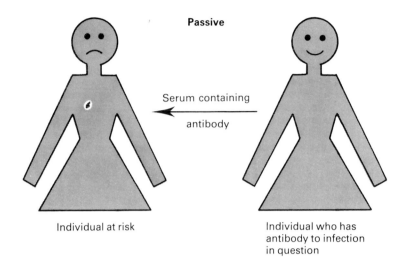

Passive

Serum containing antibody

Individual at risk

Individual who has antibody to infection in question

— Not associated with stimulation of recipient's immune response
— Acts immediately
— Short-lived

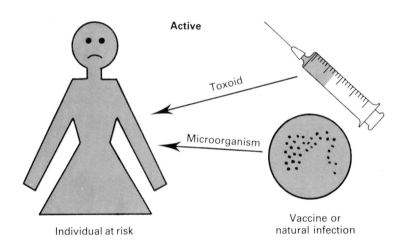

Active

Toxoid

Microorganism

Individual at risk

Vaccine or natural infection

— Results from stimulation of the individual's own immune response
— Considerable delay before protection
— Immunity long-lived— may last a lifetime

Active immunization

Active immunity results when the host mounts his *own immune response* to an antigenic stimulus. This may be acquired *naturally* following clinical or subclinical *infection* with a pathogenic organism, or *artificially* following *immunization*. The substance used for immunization must of course be safe, i.e. the pathogenic effect must be modified without losing important antigens. Vaccines may consist of *live organisms, killed organisms* or *toxoids*.

Live vaccines

Before a live organism can be administered as a vaccine, it must be *attenuated*, i.e. rendered harmless. This is most frequently achieved by growing the organism and then frequently subculturing it in the laboratory. Such propagation under unnatural conditions tends to favour the emergence of mutant strains which are not harmful to the human host.

Live vaccines produce an ongoing stimulus to the immune system due to the multiplication of the

92

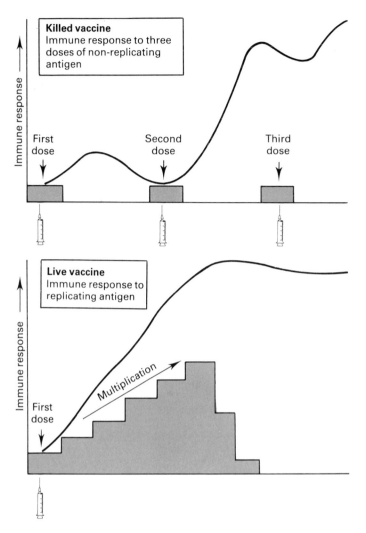

microorganism in the host. Therefore boosters are generally not required (an exception is oral polio vaccine, discussed later). A live vaccine can be ineffective if circulating antibody is already present, e.g. a patient who has already received passive immunization with immunoglobulin or a young baby who still has circulating maternal immuno-globulin. In such cases the microorganism will be rapidly destroyed before replication and adequate immunization will not therefore take place.

Side-effects of live vaccines generally take the form of a very mild infection similar to the disease against which they will protect, e.g. measles vaccine may result in a very mild attack of measles. These side-effects do not follow immediately, however, but like the natural disease manifest themselves after a variable incubation period.

Live vaccines can be dangerous in certain circum-stances. An individual who is immunosuppressed can be overcome by infection by so-called harmless attenuated organisms. LIVE VACCINES GIVEN TO AN IMMUNODEFICIENT PATIENT CAN BE LETHAL. Precautions are also necessary with pregnant women.

Killed vaccines

These vaccines are completely safe but the immun-ity conferred by them, even when given with *adjuvant*, if often inferior to that resulting from a live vaccine or natural infection. Because self-replication of the microorganism does not occur, *booster* doses of vaccine are necessary. Moreover, injected killed vaccine (e.g. cholera) may stimulate systemic antibody synthesis without initiating an adequate response in the intestine, i.e. the site of natural infection.

Toxoids

In diseases such as tetanus and diphtheria the organisms multiplying locally produce potent *exotox-ins* responsible for life-threatening effects on the heart and nervous system. These exotoxins, when purified and inactivated with formalin, are known as *toxoids* which are non-pathogenic but antigenic. When combined with an adjuvant, their administration leads to the production of *antitoxin* by the recipient.

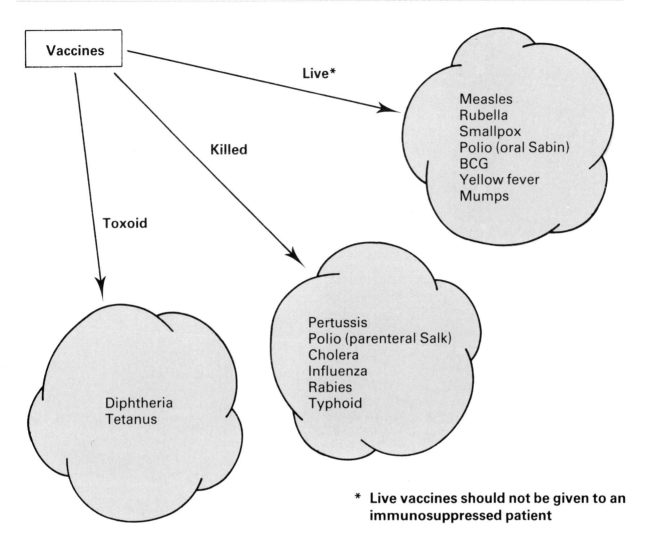

* **Live vaccines should not be given to an immunosuppressed patient**

Immunization—practical aspects

Notes on schedule

Immunization of an infant should occur during the first year of life. Theoretically, the desirable age for commencing immunization would be about 6 months because:

A. Before this age the antibody response may be reduced by the presence of maternal antibody.
B. The child's antibody forming system is immature in the early months of life.

However, schedules generally recommend the first immunization earlier than this at about 3 months. This is partly because whooping cough is a very serious illness in young children and does not seem to be prevented by maternal antibody. Early protection is therefore desirable. There is evidence that although not optimal, the immune response *can* produce significant levels of antibody *before* 6 months.

Diphtheria, tetanus, pertussis (D/T/Per or 'triple' vaccine)

Primary immunization

The first dose of this vaccine is given at the age of three months. For an optimum imune response this should be repeated after 6–8 weeks and again after 4–6 months. If pertussis immunization is contraindicated, diphtheria and tetanus (D/T) only should be given.

'Boosters'

No further immunization with pertussis is necessary. However, at school entry a further dose of D/T should be given and a dose of tetanus toxoid should be given prior to leaving school. It is advisable to give 'booster' doses of tetanus toxoid at 10-year intervals thereafter.

Recommended schedule of routine immunization in childhood

- 3–12 months
  D/T/Per or D/T
  OPV (first dose)

  6–8-week interval

  D/T/Per or D/T
  OPV (second dose)

  4–6-month interval

  D/T/Per or D/T
  OPV (third dose)

- 12–18 months (or older)
  Measles (to be replaced by MMR)

- 5–6 years (school entry)
  D/T
  OPV   booster doses

- 10–14 years (girls only)
  Rubella

  3-week interval

- 10–14 years
  BCG for the tuberculin-negative

- 15–19 years (school-leaving)
  Tetanus vaccine
  OPV

  D = diphtheria toxoid
  T = tetanus toxoid
  Per = pertussis vaccine
  OPV = oral polio vaccine

Pertussis vaccine

During the past few years there has been a marked decline in the number of infants being given this vaccine. This is largely due to much publicity regarding its possible side-effect of severe brain damage. However, the U.K. Health Department's Joint Committee of Vaccination and Immunization (1977) has concluded that the benefits of pertussis immunization outweigh the dangers. The relationship between pertussis immunization and brain damage is not clear.

As expected, the fall in numbers of vaccinated children has led to a steep rise in the number of pertussis cases. It can only be hoped that parents will continue to bring their infants for immunization against diphtheria and tetanus—if they do not, we may see the re-emergence of diphtheria in our community.

There are, however, some generally accepted contraindications to pertussis vaccine. These are:

1. A history of convulsions.
2. A family history of neonatal cerebral symptoms.
3. Acute infections—vaccination should be postponed until the child is well.

If a child has a convulsion following vaccination, no further pertussis vaccine should be given.

Poliomyelitis

In Great Britain the oral 'Sabin' vaccine is commonly used. This is a live attenuated vaccine containing types I, II and III poliovirus. Since it is given by mouth, it has the advantage of conferring some gut as well as systemic immunity. Generally three doses are given in infancy and again at school entry and on leaving school. Side-effects are very unusual.

Measles

Live attenuated vaccines are almost always used nowadays (the killed vaccines used formerly often resulted in poor immunity and untoward side-effects). A single dose of measles vaccine given in the second year of life confers a high degree of lasting protection. Occasionally immunization is followed by a mild measles-like syndrome and rarely by encephalitis (the incidence of this is probably much less than following natural measles).

Measles vaccination should be avoided in children who have:

1. A history of convulsions.
2. A history of allergy to egg.

MMR vaccine

The measles vaccine will now be replaced by a mixed mumps, measles, rubella vaccine introduced into the U.K. at the end of 1988.

BCG

This vaccine is no longer given routinely at birth in Britain, although it should be offered a few days after delivery to infants who are likely to be in contact with tuberculosis since maternal immunoglobulin is in no way protective. Normally it is offered to children aged 10–13 years who are *Mantoux*-negative. The Mantoux reaction can be temporarily suppressed during the course of viral diseases such as measles, therefore it should not be done within six weeks of such infections or immunizations.

Since BCG is a live attenuated vaccine, it is capable of causing severe, disseminated disease in immunosuppressed individuals.

Rubella

The dangers of rubella are to the foetus, particularly during the first trimester of pregnancy. It is important, therefore, that all females are immune either by natural infection or by immunization by the time they are of child-bearing age.

Vaccine is therefore offered to girls about twelve years of age. The live attenuated vaccine should *not*, however, be given *during* pregnancy since the foetus may be affected. Instead, women who are found by routine screening to be seronegative during pregnancy should be immunized in the early post-partum period.

The vaccines described above are those commonly used in Britain. Many more are available and these are described briefly on the accompanying chart.

Hepatitis B

There is increasing concern that some groups, e.g. health workers, may contract hepatitis B due to a needle stick injury or by exposure of damaged skin to the blood of a carrier.

An active vaccine prepared from pooled plasma has been available in recent years. Uptake has not been good in some areas, perhaps due to fears (which are very understandable but fortunately unfounded) that there may be a risk of contamination with the virus responsible for AIDs. No such transmission has ever been recorded.

At the time of writing a new vaccine using modern technology which does *not* depend on pooled plasma has come on to the market. This is likely to prove acceptable and should be offered to at-risk groups.

Recommended schedule of immunization of adults

• Rubella vaccine for susceptible women of childbearing age (1 dose)	A history of rubella is unreliable
	Immunization is recommended for all adult women of childbearing age who are seronegative for rubella
	Immunization should *not* take place during pregnancy
	Pregnancy must be avoided for 3 months after vaccination
• Polio vaccine for previously unvaccinated adults (3 doses)	Unvaccinated parents should receive oral polio vaccine at the same time as the first dose of oral polio vaccine is given to baby
• Active immunization against tetanus for previously unvaccinated adults (3 doses)	

Immunization in pregnancy

- Avoid all *routine** immunizations with live vaccines (e.g. rubella vaccine in pregnancy)

- Avoid killed or inactivated vaccines which commonly produce a systemic reaction

---

*Epidemics require special consideration

Immunization in pregnancy

Since live virus can cross the placenta and infect the foetus, leading to foetal abnormality or death, it should be a rule to avoid all routine immunizations with live vaccines in pregnancy. This rule includes live rubella vaccine which should *not* be given during pregnancy.

If a pregnant female requires immunization for travel purposes, a certificate of exemption is normally accepted. During an epidemic, however, the administration of live vaccine may have to be very carefully considered. Unfortunately, some killed vaccines are associated with systemic reactions. These should also if possible be avoided during pregnancy for fear of harming the foetus.

Contraindications to vaccines

1. *Pregnancy*.
2. *Immunosuppressed patients*. Live vaccines should not be given to any patient whose immune system is likely to be suppressed, e.g.
   (a) Primary immune deficiencies such as agammaglobulinaemia.
   (b) Secondary immune deficiencies such as patients receiving steroid therapy, radiotherapy, cytotoxic drugs.
   (c) Malignant disease.
   (d) Severe chronic disease.

3. *Allergic disorders*. An allergic individual may rarely have a reaction to small amounts of material present in a vaccine, e.g. theoretically, an egg sensitive patient may react to trace amounts of egg protein contaminating influenza vaccine.
4. *Poor health*. Normally vaccination should occur when a patient is in optimal health. This helps ensure that a maximum immune response will be obtained from the vaccine and protection should result.

Tetanus

Tetanus is an extremely serious condition caused by a potent neurotoxin produced by the organism *Clostridium tetani*. Even with modern intensive care facilities mortality from the condition is still between 12 and 30%.

It is important to realize that tetanus is not spread by human to human contact, therefore vaccination schedules which lead to large numbers of the population being immune do not lead to a reduction in the numbers of *Cl. tetani* in the community. The organism does not need the human host to survive—it is present in the soil, hence farmers, gardeners and sportsmen who are not immunized are continually at risk.

Although immunization schedules ensure that almost all babies are fully protected, and boosting doses are given during schooldays, this has not always been the case. Indeed it should be assumed that anyone over the age of 50 is unprotected.

It should always be remembered also that even apparently trivial wounds can result in tetanus. There may be no evidence that the wound is infected, e.g. an elderly female pricking herself while pruning roses could be at risk.

The following types of wound should be considered 'high risk'. The important factor is that they all have a poor blood supply:

1. Wounds containing damaged dead tissue.
2. Deep, contused wounds.
3. Wounds containing foreign bodies.
4. Wounds contaminated with soil, grit.
5. Wounds already infected with other organisms.
6. Puncture wounds.
7. Wounds in areas of the body where blood supply is poor, e.g. foot, lower leg. This is particularly true in the elderly or diabetic patient.

When a patient presents with a wound in one of the above 'at-risk' categories, the procedure should be as follows:

A. *Surgical debridement*

Thorough surgical toilet of all wounds, regardless of how trivial, should be performed.

B. *Find out when the wound occurred*

If the wound does not come into the above 'at-risk' categories and is less than 6 hours old, surgical toilet generally will provide sufficient prophylaxis against tetanus.

C. *Enquire about patient's immune status*

If the patient has had no previous tetanus toxoid, has had an incomplete course, has had no 'boosters' over the previous 10 years, or the immune status is unknown, consider PASSIVE immunization with human anti-tetanus immunoglobulin. This should be given in patients with dirty, neglected, penetrating wounds. If more than 24 hours have elapsed since the wound was sustained, or if there is a very high risk of contamination with *Cl. tetani*, passive immunization should be given REGARDLESS OF PREVIOUS IMMUNIZATION HISTORY.

D. *Consider antibiotic therapy*

E. *Consider active immunization with tetanus toxoid*

It is extremely unlikely that antibody will reach protective levels after a first injection of tetanus toxoid in a previously unprotected individual. However, active vaccination should be commenced in all patients who have received human anti-tetanus immunoglobulin passively and the primary course should be completed. This will protect them from the risk in subsequent injuries. If a previously fully immunized individual has received a dose of tetanus toxoid within the previous year, no further boosting is necessary. If the last booster was more than one year previously one dose of booster should be given.

Vaccines not routinely used in UK
– used by travellers or others at particular risk

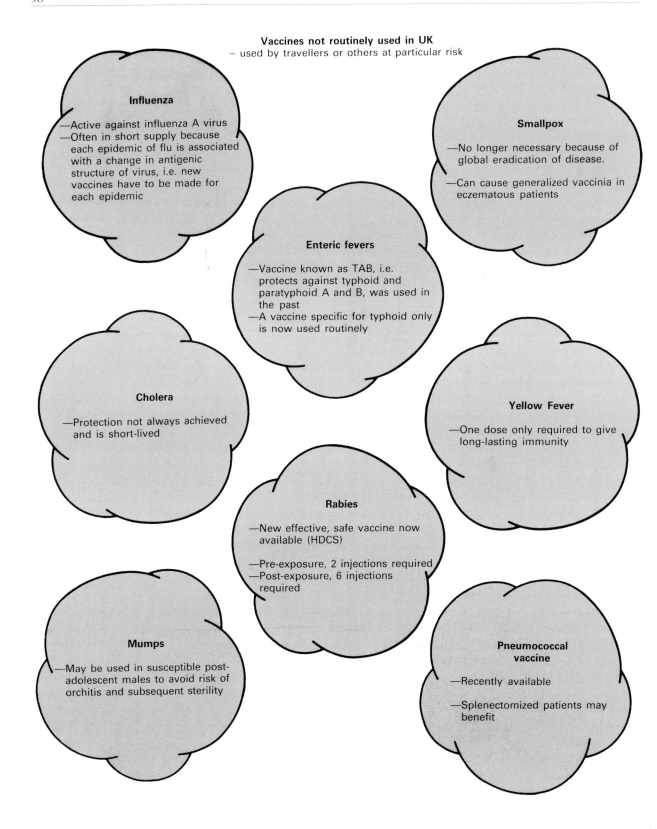

Influenza

—Active against influenza A virus
—Often in short supply because
each epidemic of flu is associated
with a change in antigenic
structure of virus, i.e. new
vaccines have to be made for
each epidemic

Smallpox

—No longer necessary because of
global eradication of disease.

—Can cause generalized vaccinia in
eczematous patients

Enteric fevers

—Vaccine known as TAB, i.e.
protects against typhoid and
paratyphoid A and B, was used in
the past
—A vaccine specific for typhoid only
is now used routinely

Cholera

—Protection not always achieved
and is short-lived

Yellow Fever

—One dose only required to give
long-lasting immunity

Rabies

—New effective, safe vaccine now
available (HDCS)

—Pre-exposure, 2 injections required
—Post-exposure, 6 injections
required

Mumps

—May be used in susceptible post-
adolescent males to avoid risk of
orchitis and subsequent sterility

**Pneumococcal
vaccine**

—Recently available

—Splenectomized patients may
benefit

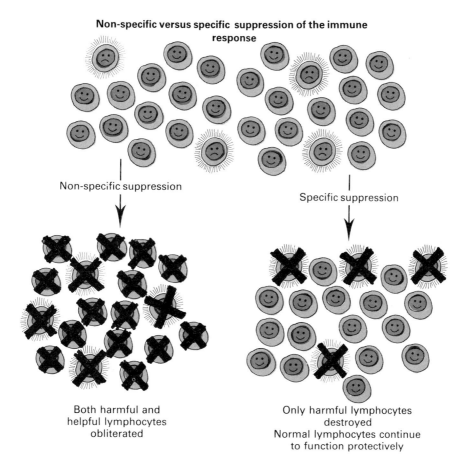

Non-specific versus specific suppression of the immune response

Non-specific suppression

Specific suppression

Both harmful and
helpful lymphocytes
obliterated

Only harmful lymphocytes
destroyed
Normal lymphocytes continue
to function protectively

19. Immunosuppression

As discussed previously, the immune response can on certain occasions be harmful to the host—sometimes so harmful that severe and perhaps even fatal disease may result. In these circumstances a reasonable therapeutic approach is to 'dampen down' the immune response using *immunosuppressive agents*.

Conditions where immunosuppressive therapy is useful

1. *Autoimmune disease*, e.g. disseminated lupus erythematosus.
2. *Hypersensitivity states*, e.g. immune complex glomerulonephritis.
3. *Transplantation*, e.g. to prevent rejection of transplanted kidney.
4. *Tumours*—in this case drugs are used to destroy the malignant cell but unfortunately cells of the immune system are also damaged to a greater or lesser extent, leading to depression of the immune response.

Non-specific versus specific suppression of the immune response

Non-specific immunosuppression is a crude unselective generalized suppression of all or many of the body's immune responses. Unfortunately, the responses that are beneficial to the host are also suppressed, resulting in a markedly increased vulnerability to infection. This, unfortunately, is the method of immunosuppression that we have to rely on mainly until now.

Specific immunosuppression is a much more sophisticated method of immunosuppression and is the ultimate aim. Here, only the immune response to the harmful antigen is suppressed, with conservation of the protective immune responses to unrelated antigens. Unfortunately, medical knowledge is not yet at the stage where we are widely able to use this method of immunosuppression in a therapeutic manner. Theoretically, such immunosuppression would not result in an increased risk of infection which is so often seen with the methods currently in use.

Immunosuppression

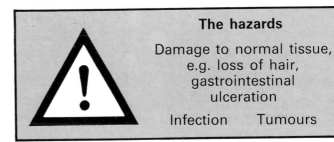

Methods used	The hazards
X-rays Cytotoxic drugs Antilymphocytic serum	Damage to normal tissue, e.g. loss of hair, gastrointestinal ulceration Infection Tumours

Immunosuppression—the crude methods of today

Methods of inducing non-specific immunosuppression

Removal of lymphoid cells or lymphoid organs

Theoretically, removal of large numbers of circulating lymphocytes or removal of lymphoid organs would result in immunosuppression. These procedures have very little place in the management of human conditions.

X-rays

This was one of the first methods of immunosuppression to be used therapeutically. X-rays prevent DNA synthesis in lymphocytes and their precursors, leading to failure of replication of these cells following exposure.

Cytotoxic drugs

This is the method most commonly used nowadays to suppress the immune response. These drugs fall into various groups depending on their mode of action.

A. *Steroids* (e.g. hydrocortisone, prednisolone) have a suppressive effect on polymorphs and macrophages as well as antibody production.
B. *Antimetabolites* (e.g. azathioprine, 6-mercaptopurine, methotrexate) have a chemical structure very similar but not identical to enzyme substrates in the body. They therefore compete for binding sites on enzyme molecules and prevent certain necessary biochemical reactions.
C. *Alkylating agents* (e.g. cyclophosphamide) interfere with nucleic acid synthesis.

Immunosuppressive drugs generally act more efficiently on rapidly dividing cells than on normal cells, hence, as well as having an effect on lymphocytes, they also are very effective on proliferating tumour cells. Most of these drugs are therefore also regarded as antitumour agents.

Although the aim is to destroy rapidly dividing cells, normal cells are almost always damaged to a lesser degree during the course of *cytotoxic therapy*. This is manifest clinically as, for example, oral or gastrointestinal ulceration, loss of hair.

Antibodies

Since lymphocytes are responsible for the damaging effects of the immune response, a possible way of destroying them but leaving the other cells of the body intact might be to raise an antibody against human lymphocytes. This *antiserum* could then be injected into the patient and destroy his lymphocytes.

This method was used mainly in the attempt to prevent rejection of renal grafts. T lymphocytes are more important in rejection processes than B lymphocytes. Antibody can be prepared by injecting human T lymphocytes into horses. These lymphocytes are recognized as foreign by the animal, and antibody against human T lymphocytes is produced. Horse serum containing this antibody can then be purified and injected into the patient. Such serum is known as *antilymphocytic globulin* (ALG). Hopefully, T lymphocytes would be destroyed while B lymphocytes remain intact.

Unfortunately antilymphocytic globulin is a foreign protein (horse gammaglobulin) and the recipient can suffer severe hypersensitivity reactions as his own body recognizes it as foreign.

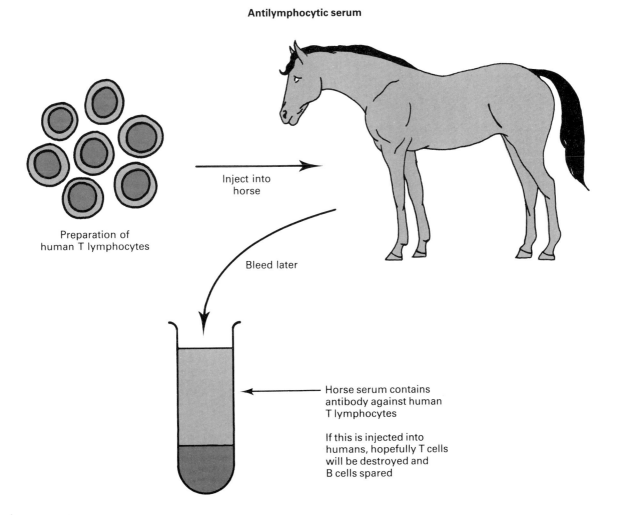

Antilymphocytic serum

Preparation of human T lymphocytes

Inject into horse

Bleed later

Horse serum contains antibody against human T lymphocytes

If this is injected into humans, hopefully T cells will be destroyed and B cells spared

Non-specific immunosuppression—the hazards

Infection

The immune response to most infectious agents is suppressed during the course of immunosuppressive therapy as it is used today. Hence, *recurrent* or *severe infection* with all the common pathogens and also severe infection with the patient's own (normally harmless) bacterial flora occurs frequently. Indeed, no organism can safely be regarded as *non-pathogenic* in a patient who is severely immunosuppressed.

Tumours

It has been observed that there has been an increased incidence of cancer in patients undergoing immunosuppressive therapy. This may be the result of depression of T lymphocytes which seem to have an important role in *immunological surveillance* against emerging malignant cells.

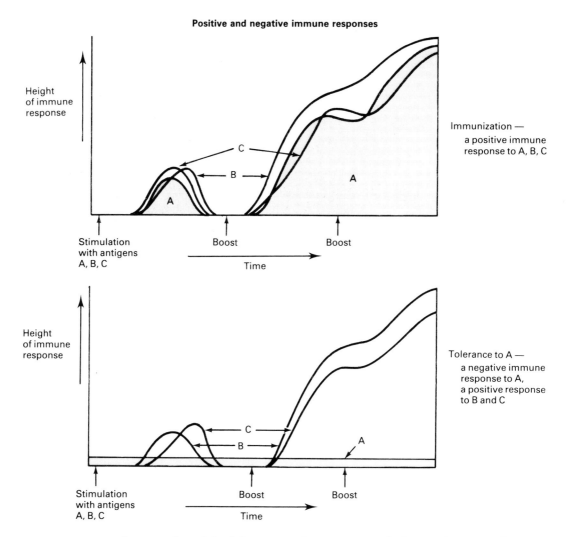

Positive and negative immune responses

Height of immune response

C

B

A

A

Immunization —
a positive immune
response to A, B, C

Stimulation
with antigens
A, B, C

Boost

Boost

Time

Height
of immune
response

C

B

A

Tolerance to A —
a negative immune
response to A,
a positive response
to B and C

Stimulation
with antigens
A, B, C

Boost

Boost

Time

Immunosuppression—the highly specific methods of tomorrow

Cyclosporin-A

This is an immunosuppressive agent which has been used to prevent transplant rejection.

It is much more specific than the others, acting predominantly on certain subclasses of T lymphocytes during their early phases of cell division. Resting T lymphocytes remain unaffected and there is little toxicity for non-lymphocytic cells, e.g. those lining the gastrointestinal tract. Serum levels of the drug have to be carefully monitored, however, because of nephrotoxicity.

Because of its selective nature, it represents a very significant advance in immunosuppressive therapy.

Immunological tolerance

Once we fully understand the mechanisms involved in the phenomenon known as *immunological*

tolerance we may be in a position to induce exquisitely specific immunosuppression free from the side-effects normally associated with generalized immuno-suppression.

What is meant by immunological tolerance? When an individual mounts an immune response against a given antigen, one generally thinks in terms of a very specific reaction involving both T and B cells which is *positive* in nature and results ultimately in the elimination of the offending antigen. However, this is not always the case. Sometimes the immune response can be a *negative* but nonetheless specific phenomenon against a certain antigen, i.e. in some way the immune response is *stimulated* by an antigen *not* to react against it when it meets it subsequently. Such a phenomenon is known as *immunological tolerance*. This negative response to an antigen is much less well understood than the more familiar positive response of immunization. However, the phenomenon has very considerable implications in the future management of patients with immunological problems.

Factors involved in production of tolerance

Antigen factors
The dose
The route
The chemical
configuration

Host factors
Immunological
immaturity
Type of lymphocyte
stimulated

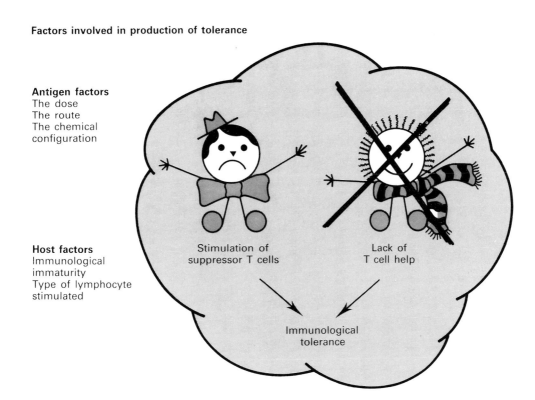

Stimulation of
suppressor T cells

Lack of
T cell help

Immunological
tolerance

Self versus non-self

Mechanisms of *tolerance* are probably responsible for the fact that normally we do not produce an immune response against our own body constituents. Some interesting observations relevant to this have been made in twin calves. As in humans there are two types of twins:

1. *Identical twins*—These twins are genetically identical, i.e. the antigenic structure of their constituents is the same. One twin, therefore, will recognize the other twin as self and an immune reaction will not be mounted.
2. *Non-identical twins*—These twins are no more similar than brother and sister and normally the body constituents of one twin will be recognized by the other as foreign and an immune response will result.

However, sometimes in calves the phenomenon of *chimerism* is observed. This means that non-identical twins have an anastomosis of some of the blood vessels of their placenta, hence during foetal life they have shared their circulations, i.e. twin A during foetal life has been exposed to the blood cells of twin B and vice versa. In these circumstances the twins after birth recognize each other as self, i.e. each is immunologically tolerant of the other's antigens. This is because it appears that in foetal life all antigens met are recognized as self and the immune system is programmed not to react against them.

What causes tolerance rather than the more familiar positive immune response?

The factors that decide that a negative response results rather than a positive one are poorly understood. However, the following appear to be important.

Antigen factors

The dose—Very small doses and very high doses of antigen seem able to induce a negative response. Intermediate dosage leads to positive immunization.

The route—Repeated oral administration of some antigens may be more liable to produce tolerance than, for example, intramuscular administration. This may be important in preventing hypersensitivity reactions to the food that we eat.

The chemical configuration—In general, tolerance is more easily induced with simple antigens than with complicated substances that have many *antigenic determinants*.

Host factors

Immunological immaturity—Tolerance can be more easily induced in the young immature animal than in the adult.

Lymphocyte stimulation—It is very likely that tolerance is induced and maintained by stimulation of *specific suppressor T cells* which act by 'turning off' a specific immune response to a given antigen while leaving other immune responses intact. If for any reason suppressor T cells are insufficient or not able to be stimulated, tolerance to some 'self antigens' may be lost and autoimmune disease may result.

If at this stage you feel you do not really understand the mechanisms involved in tolerance, do not despair—not many immunologists understand them either! However, a total understanding of the mechanisms will come some day and following this we may see one of the biggest breakthroughs in immunology—the ability to manipulate the immune response in such a way as to suppress only the immune responses of one's choice while leaving the others intact. Edward Jenner in his vaccination against smallpox did after all manage to do this therapeutically in a positive way about 180 years ago. It is frustrating that we have not yet been able to do the same thing in a negative way in the twentieth century!

Section C
AIDS—acquired immunodeficiency syndrome

20. The background

The 1980s will undoubtedly be remembered historically as the decade during which AIDS took the world by surprise. Immunologically, it heralded a new era. Until then, 'acquired immunodeficiency' undoubtedly existed—but in an entirely different context. Almost invariably it was associated with *medical advancement*. For example, tissue transplantation, anti-tumour therapy and the management of some autoimmune diseases all shared the same common iatrogenic side-effect to a greater or lesser extent: suppression of the immune response.

In the summer months of 1981, however, it became clear in the U.S.A. that the clinical features of a severe acquired immune deficiency were appearing in young men who had no history of ever having received immunosuppressive medical therapy. Indeed, the men had been previously in good health. They were, however, all homosexual.

How AIDS presented itself

Fortunately, many countries have an 'early warning system' where individual cases of infectious and other medical conditions are reported. The 'powerhouse' for this operation in the U.S.A. is at the Centers for Disease Control (CDC) in Atlanta, Georgia. Such centres are very aware of the normal 'background' prevalence of various medical conditions within a country. When increased numbers of patients with a given condition are reported, or if clustering occurs within a particular area of a country, the staff in such centres can identify this immediately. Lines of communication are then set up nationally and if necessary internationally to ensure that further cases are quickly identified and preventative measures are put into effect as quickly as possible.

The reporting of two unusual conditions to the CDC in Atlanta heralded the onset of the AIDS epidemic. The first were reports of pneumonia caused by the organism *Pneumocystis carinii* and the other of a tumour: *Kaposi's sarcoma*. By the winter of 1981 more than 150 cases had been reported. Both conditions occurred in homosexual and bisexual men who had previously been healthy. There were clusters in three American cities: New York, San Francisco and Los Angeles.

Pneumocystis carinii pneumonia had until that time been associated with immune suppression usually involving the cell-mediated limb of the immune response. When these men were investigated it was confirmed that they did indeed suffer from a severe defect of cellular immunity. In the early days, the cause of this deficiency was unclear. However, the clustering of cases suggested that an infective agent may be involved and the type of patient suggested that the mode of spread was likely to be venereal.

In 1983, the causal agent was identified. This has been given various names over the past few years (see diagram); however, it has now been agreed internationally that the virus should be known as *human immunodeficiency virus (HIV)*.

Some AIDS terminology

AIDS	Acquired immunodeficiency syndrome
HIV	Human immunodeficiency virus (2 types: HIV-1 and HIV-2)
HTLV-III*	Human T lymphotropic virus type III
LAV*	Lymphadenopathy-associated virus
ARV*	AIDS-associated retrovirus
ARC	AIDS-related complex
PGL	Persistent generalized lymphadenopathy
STD	Sexually transmitted disease
CDC	Centres for disease control
WHO	World Health Organization
PCP	*Pneumcystis carinii* pneumonia
KS	Kaposis sarcoma
CMV	Cytomegalovirus
EBV	Epstein–Barr virus
HSV	Herpes simplex virus
PML	Progressive multifocal leucoencephalopathy
VSV	Varicella zoster virus
T_4 cells	T-lymphocytes with helper function. Previously known as OKT4 cells. Now known as CD4 cells.
T_8 cells	T-lymphocytes exhibiting suppressor/cytotoxic function. Previously known as OKT8 cells. Now known as CD8 cells.

*All former names for HIV.

Mode of transmission of the virus

Although the first patients reported were homosexuals, it has now become clear that AIDS is not exclusively a venereal disease. Soon afterwards, other 'at-risk' groups were identified. These groups included intravenous drug abusers, recipients of blood and blood products, individuals who had in some way been associated with parts of Africa and heterosexual partners of AIDS patients. In the early days, being Haitian was also considered a risk factor, but this is no longer the case.

AIDS—At-risk groups

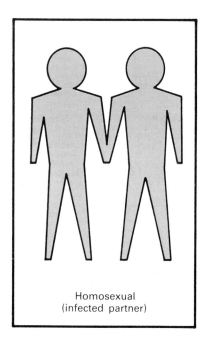

Homosexual
(infected partner)

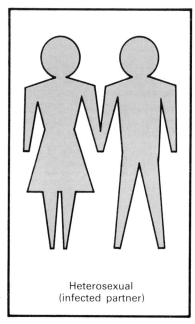

Heterosexual
(infected partner)

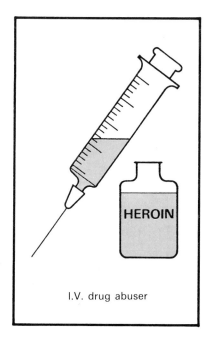

I.V. drug abuser

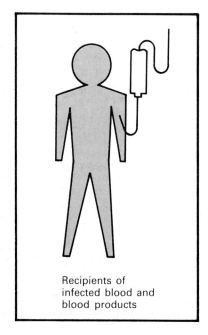

Recipients of
infected blood and
blood products

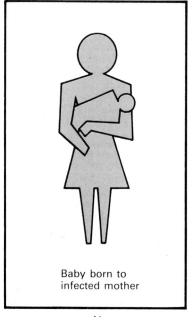

Baby born to
infected mother

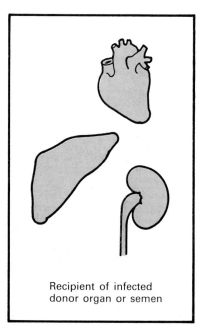

Recipient of infected
donor organ or semen

Also
A minimal risk from accidental exposure

How and where did the virus originate?

This question has not yet been fully answered and various theories have been proposed.

Haiti is a popular holiday resort of homosexuals in the U.S.A. There was a high prevalence of Haitians among the first AIDS cases reported. This led to the wrong conclusion that Haiti was the country of origin of the disease.

It is now apparent that the disease originated in Central Africa. Indeed, there is evidence of infection with the virus in African serum which had been stored since the mid-1970s. The Haitian connection seems to result from migrant Africans settling in the Caribbean. Homosexual holidaymakers from the U.S.A. then contracted the virus following sexual exposure. On returning home, the virus spread like wildfire throughout the homosexual population in certain American cities, largely as a result of the large numbers of homosexual partners of each Haitian contact.

The subsequent spread of the virus

The number of new AIDS cases in the U.S.A. has increased relentlessly since 1981 and cases have now been reported from every state. A convenient way to estimate the rate of spread is to calculate the time taken for the number of reported cases to double. Initially, the doubling time was five months, indicating rapid spread of the disease. In New York and California there is evidence that the 'doubling time' is lengthening. Hopefully, this trend will continue elsewhere.

While the disease was spreading throughout the 'at-risk' population in the United States, cases were being reported from most of Europe. Spread within these countries tended to mimic what had already happened in the United States a few years before. Outside Europe, Russia and the Far East have had no problem until very recently, but the disease is now appearing in these countries also. It is likely that every country is now affected. Reports are now

The probable origin and spread of AIDS

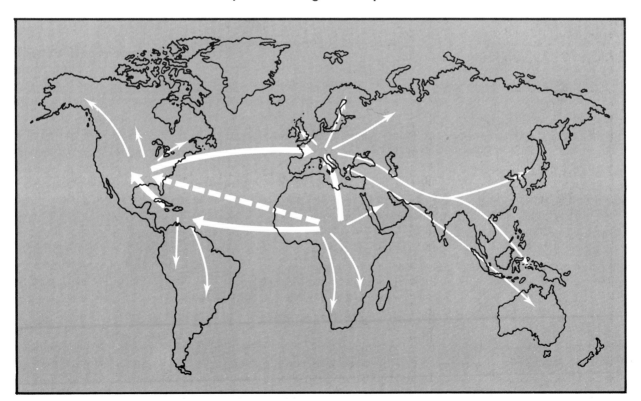

collaborated by the World Health Organization at a special headquarters in Paris.

Worldwide, homosexual men accounted for the highest proportion of AIDS cases. They were responsible for approximately 65% of cases in the U.S.A. and 88% of cases in Britain in March 1987. This is followed by intravenous drug abusers in the U.S.A. (approx. 17%). At present in Britain there are more haemophiliacs with frank AIDS than there are i.v. drug abusers. This figure is likely to change in the near future, however, since in some parts of Britain there is a very worrying spread of the virus among drug addicts, only a few of whom have as yet developed AIDS.

AIDS in Africa

In Africa, the picture is entirely different. There, AIDS affects both men and women equally. The heterosexual nature of the disease there appears to be related to sexual promiscuity and a high level of prostitution within the areas most affected. Because a high proportion of the population carry the virus, spread via blood transfusion and the use of contaminated needles is also important.

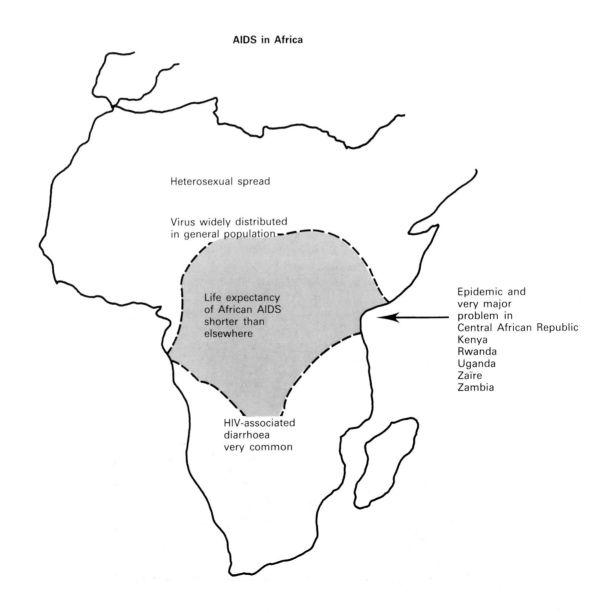

AIDS in Africa

Heterosexual spread

Virus widely distributed in general population

Life expectancy of African AIDS shorter than elsewhere

HIV-associated diarrhoea very common

Epidemic and very major problem in
Central African Republic
Kenya
Rwanda
Uganda
Zaïre
Zambia

21. The spectrum of disease caused by HIV

Most epidemiological figures quote the number of cases reported suffering from the signs and symptoms of AIDS. However, many more people are infected with the virus but at present show no evidence of disease.

Whether an individual can become infected with HIV and remain completely symptom-free until old age is not yet known. There are some disconcerting studies, however, which show that with the passage of time many symptomless carriers go on to develop frank AIDS. In a retrospective study in the U.S.A., in a group of homosexual men showing serological evidence of infection with the virus in 1980 only 1 in 800 had frank AIDS. However, in 1986, this ratio had decreased to 1 in 15. Not all observations are as pessimistic as this, however, and the long-term results of many more prospective studies are awaited.

It is now known that there are several disease patterns, ranging from the asymptomatic carrier to the patient with frank AIDS. In 1986 CDC produced a classification system for HIV infections. The older classification and newer classification are shown in the accompanying diagrams.

Previous classification of HIV infections

- The seroconversion illness
- Healthy carriers
- Persistent generalized lymphadenopathy
- AIDS-related complex
- AIDS

Current classification of HIV infection

Group I	Acute infection
Group II	Asymptomatic infection
Group III	Persistent generalized lymphadenopathy
Group IV	Other disease
Subgroup A	Constitutional disease
Subgroup B	Neurological disease
Subgroup C	Secondary infectious diseases
Category C1	Specified secondary infectious diseases listed in the CDC surveillance definition for AIDS
Category C2	Other specified secondary infectious diseases
Subgroup D	Secondary cancers
Subgroup E	Other conditions

Acute infection (classified as group I)

As with other infectious diseases, when an individual meets the causal organism the immune system responds. This response can be measured soon afterwards by detecting specific antibody to the infecting agent. When an individual is first infected with HIV, he sometimes suffers an acute illness similar to glandular fever immediately before antibody to HIV can be detected in his blood. This is known as the *seroconversion illness*. Patients are considered particularly infectious during this stage. The range of symptoms associated with seroconversion is wide, ranging from a mild flu-like illness to a severe meningitis or encephalitis (see diagram). The majority of patients, however, are asymptomatic during this period.

Definition of acute HIV infection
Group I

A mononucleosis-like syndrome, with or without aseptic meningitis, associated with seroconversion for HIV antibody
(Antibody seroconversion is required as evidence of initial infection. Current procedures for viral isolation are not adequately sensitive to be relied on for demonstrating infection onset)

Symptoms and signs sometimes associated with the seroconversion illness

A 'glandular fever-like' syndrome

- Sudden onset
- Fever and sweats
- Tiredness and malaise
- Nausea and anorexia
- Muscle and joint aches
- Headaches
- Sore throat
- Diarrhoea
- Transient rash
- Generalized lymphadenopathy
- Atypical lymphocytosis
- Seroconversion generally follows in 3–8 weeks
- Syndrome resolves spontaneously
- Lasts 3–14 days

> ## Definition of asymptomatic HIV infection
> ## Group II
>
> The absence of symptoms or signs of HIV infection in a patient known to be Antibody-positive
> If a patient has previous symptoms or signs that would have placed him in group III or IV he cannot be replaced in Group II

Asymptomatic HIV infection (classified as group II)

By definition, these patients are infected with HIV and yet experience no symptoms or signs. Some may become symptomatic within a few months and others may remain symptom-free for many years, perhaps for decades. What the future holds for them in the long term is not yet known.

A subgroup of these patients will demonstrate abnormalities of immune function (see later). Whether they are at risk of becoming symptomatic sooner rather than later is not known but this is currently being closely looked at in ongoing prospective studies.

At the present time, *all* of these asymptomatic patients should be regarded as every bit as infectious (perhaps even more so) as the patient suffering from frank AIDS.

Persistent generalized lymphadenopathy (PGL, classified as group III)

Most patients in this group are symptom-free and may remain so for many years. Lymph node biopsy shows benign reactive hyperplasia. In some, the lymphadenopathy may resolve and the patients become asymptomatic carriers. They should *not* be reclassified into group II, however.

Some patients develop constitutional symptoms. This often heralds progression of the disease to group IV. The proportion of patients with PGL who will progress to frank AIDS is not yet known. Several prospective studies are ongoing but the results so far are variable. It may be that certain types of patients are more prone than others to develop the full-blown syndrome owing to intercurrent and apparently unrelated events (see later).

> ## Definition of persistent generalized lymphadenopathy (PGL)
>
> Palpable lymhadenopathy (lymph node enlargement of 1 cm or greater) at two or more extrainguinal sites persisting for more than 3 months in the absence of a concurrent illness or condition other than HIV infection to explain the findings

Other disease (classified as group IV)

This group of patients may or may not have lymphadenopathy in addition to other clinical features of HIV infection. Classification into group IV depends on the *type* of symptom, *not* its severity.

Constitutional disease (classified as group IV, subgroup A)

Sometimes a patient may demonstrate some of the generalized symptoms usually found in patients with full-blown AIDS but show no evidence of opportunistic infections or tumours.

Formerly patients in this group would have been considered to be suffering from *AIDS-related complex* (*ARC*). This term was rather 'looser' than the present definition and should now be avoided. It is likely to be referred to in the medical literature, however, for some time, and so for completeness the definition has been summarized in the accompanying diagram.

Definition of constitutional disease Group IV subgroup A

One or more of the following:
- Fever persisting more than one month
- Involuntary weight loss of greater than 10% of baseline
- Diarrhoea persisting more than 1 month

In the absence of a concurrent illness or condition other than HIV infection to explain the findings

---

Features of AIDS-related complex (ARC)

Clinical Features
- Chronic diarrhoea
- Pyrexia of unknown origin for 2 months
- Tiredness and malaise
- Weight loss
- Minor oral infections, e.g. herpes and *Candida*
- Persistent generalized lymphadenopathy
- Hairy leucoplakia
- Hepatosplenomegaly

Laboratory features
- HIV antibody positive
- HIV isolation
- Lymphopenia
- T helper depression
- Elevated immunoglobulins
- Anaemia
- Thrombocytopenia
- Elevated ESR

Neurological disease (group IV, subgroup B)

Dementia

A proportion of patients with frank AIDS suffer from opportunistic infections or tumours which may cause neurological symptoms and signs. However, HIV infection *per se* can be responsible for disease of the nervous system. It is this type of patient who is classified within subgroup B. The condition is known as *AIDS dementia complex* and probably affects most patients with AIDS, often as a terminal event.

About 25% of patients who develop symptoms of AIDS dementia complex have no history of opportunistic infection or tumours and therefore cannot be truly classified as suffering from AIDS. The majority, however, demonstrate some evidence of constitutional disease or generalized lymphadeno-pathy. A small minority develop dementia who are otherwise asymptomatic, and death can occur before the appearance of any other complications.

In the early stages of AIDS, dementia may only present itself in small ways and may be missed on clinical examination. The patient may complain of difficulty in concentrating or of mild memory impairment. As the condition progresses, he becomes apathetic and socially withdrawn. Later, agitation, hallucinations, and confusion appear and in the terminal stages the patient may be bed-ridden and incapable of any communication.

It appears that AIDS dementia complex is the result of direct infection of the brain by HIV. Viral antigen has been detected in the brain and cerebrospinal fluid of these patients.

As yet it is unknown whether with the passage of time AIDS dementia will appear as a late manifestation of HIV carriers who have for many years been asymptomatic.

**Definition of neurological disease
Group IV subgroup B**

One or more of the following:

- Dementia
- Myelopathy
- Peripheral neuropathy

In the absence of a concurrent illness or condition other than HIV to explain the findings

Secondary infectious diseases (classified as group IV, subgroup C)

This classification is used to define these patients known to be infected with HIV who are also suffering or have suffered from *another* infectious disease. This secondary infection must be one that is usually associated with a defect in cell-mediated immunity.

The patients are further grouped into either category C1 or C2, depending on *which type* of infectious disease has been diagnosed.

Category C1 infections

- *Pneumocystis carinii* pneumonia
- Chronic cryptosporidiosis
- Toxoplasmosis
- Extraintestinal strongyloidiasis
- Isosporiasis
- Candidiasis (oesophageal, bronchial or pulmonary)
- Cryptococcosis
- Histoplasmosis
- Infection with *mycobacterium avium* or *Mycobacterium Kansasii*
- Cytomegalovirus infection
- Chronic mucocutaneous or disseminated herpes simplex virus infection
- Progressive multifocal leukoencephalopathy

Category C2 infections

- Oral hairy leukoplakia
- Multidermatomal herpes zoster
- Recurrent salmonella bacteraemia
- Nocardiosis
- Tuberculosis
- Oral candidiasis

Category C1 infections only are included in the definition of AIDS

**List of cancers associated with HIV infection
Group IV subgroup D**

- Kaposi's sarcoma
- Non-Hodgkin's lymphoma (small, non-cleaved lymphoma or immunoblastic sarcoma)
- Primary lymphoma of the brain

Secondary cancers (classified as group IV, subgroup D)

As well as certain infections being associated with defects in cell-mediated immunity, so also are certain tumours. Kaposi's sarcoma was the first of these to be recognized in AIDS patients, but others are now firmly associated with HIV infection.

Other conditions seen in patients with HIV infection (classified as group IV, subgroup E)

This classification is used for a patient who is infected with HIV and who is suffering from some other condition that is not classified in the groups above.

The coexisting condition may clearly be associated with immune deficiency or may not. It may be a totally unrelated clinical illness and the course and management of this may be complicated by the coexistence of HIV infection.

Notes on the current classification system

1. Much has still to be learned about HIV infection. Because of this it is likely that the current classification system outlined above will require to be changed from time to time as new information becomes available.
2. Group IV, subgroup E may appear to be a general rag-bag. It does, however, serve a very useful purpose. By recording any disease entity, however apparently unrelated to disorders of the immune system, in patients who are HIV infected, trends, associations, and problems will become evident. Some conditions presently within this group will possibly become firmly linked with AIDS or PGL in the future and be transferred into different groups or subgroups.
3. Group I is a temporary classification. It only describes patients who have transient symptoms and signs of acute infection. Following recovery, the patient will then be classified into groups II–IV depending on his subsequent symptoms or lack of them.
4. A patient, once classified as group IV, cannot revert to group III or group II even if he apparently recovers totally. Similarly, a patient who has PGL (group III) cannot revert to group II even if the lymphadenopathy resolves completely.
5. The subgroups within group IV are not mutually exclusive. An individual may for example have infections, tumours and dementia and be classified as group IV, subgroup B, C1, and D.

Which patients with HIV infection suffer from AIDS?

In 1981, a formal definition was used by CDC for the purpose of national reporting of the disease. The new classification in no way alters this definiion.

Definition of AIDS

A person is considered to have AIDS if:

A. He has a reliably diagnosed disease at least moderately indicative of an underlying cellular immune deficiency, e.g. Kaposi's sarcoma in a patient aged less than 60 years, or an opportunistic infection.*
B. He has no known underlying cause of cellular immune deficiency or any other cause of reduced resistance reported to be associated with the disease.

Once the virus was isolated, another clause was added to the 1981 definition:

C. Patients are excluded from the diagnosis of AIDS if they are anti-HIV negative and have normal T helper lymphocyte counts.

It can be seen then, that patients classified within group IV, subgroup C1, and group IV, subgroup D are those who suffer from AIDS. Some AIDS patients may also have clinical features which assign them, in addition, to another subgroup of group IV.

*These are the diseases listed on p. 116 and above.

22. Virological and immunological features of AIDS

Retroviruses

When the full impact of the clinical features of AIDS became clear, immunologists recognized that the picture was that of a cell-mediated deficiency. Virologists too had some important observations to make. Clinically, AIDS demonstrated some of the features of viral diseases which had been observed in various animals since the turn of the century. For instance, it was known that leukaemia and other tumours could be transferred in chickens owing to infection with a particular type of virus. Breast tumours could be passed from mouse to mouse and immune deficiency and leukaemia could be transferred in cats. In each case the malignancy and/or immune deficiency were due to a family of very unusual viruses known as *retroviruses*. In the late 1970s it became evident that a particular type of retrovirus could cause leukaemia in *humans*. This involved T lymphocytes.

Was AIDS due then to a new type of virus? This proved to be the case. In 1983 a new retrovirus was isolated in Paris from a patient with persistent generalized lymphadenopathy. It was named 'lymphadenopathy associated virus' (LAV) by the Paris research group. A year later an American group isolated a retrovirus from patients with AIDS. They named it 'human T cell lymphotropic virus, type III' (HTLV-III) because of its similarities to the two types of retrovirus HTLV-I and HTLV-II which had been discovered a few years previously. It soon became clear that the virus LAV and HTLV-III were indeed the same and were quite definitely the cause of AIDS. In the present state of our knowledge it appears it is a *new virus* which probably appeared in sub-Saharan Africa for the first time some 10–15 years before its first isolation.

There have been problems in accurately classifying the virus. Although initially thought to be closely related to the other human retroviruses HTLV-I and HTLV-II, recent work has linked it more closely with another retrovirus which causes inflammation of the central nervous system in sheep. This is known as the Visna virus. It is significant that with the passage of time, one important aspect of AIDS that is emerging is the effect on the central nervous system. The virus responsible for AIDS has therefore now been placed along with Visna virus into the subfamily of retroviruses known as *lentiviruses*. It has been renamed *human immunodeficiency virus* (HIV). Hopefully, this will remain its permanent name and further confusing nomenclature will be avoided!

The relationship between HIV and T lymphocytes

T lymphocytes consist of several subgroups. The T helper lymphocyte has a crucial role to play. It activates other lymphocytes, preparing them to attack foreign agents such as viruses, bacteria and tumour cells which may be harmful to the host. The helper lymphocyte therefore 'switches on' a very large part of the immune system. Without it, the other cells of the system circulate the body undirected and oblivious to danger. T helper lymphocytes are often referred to as T4 cells because they have a structure on their surface known as the T4 receptor.

Human immunodeficiency virus has a particular affinity for helper lymphocytes. It recognizes the T4 receptor on the cell and attaches itself to this. It then enters the cell and incorporates its genetic material into that of the host lymphocyte. At this stage the virus can be regarded as being out of reach. Sooner or later, however, the T cell which is infected with HIV will be stimulated into activity, perhaps due to another type of infection, and the genetic material of the HIV within the T lymphocyte takes advantage of the situation. It begins to replicate, producing young viruses which bud and separate from the 'adopted parent' T cell. Hence another generation of viruses are produced which further attack T4 lymphocytes. And so the sequence continues until most of the patient's helper cells have resident HIV or are killed by the infective process.

It is likely that some virally infected T cells are recognized by healthy cells of the immune system as foreign and in an attempt to eradicate infection are destroyed. This, however, exacerbates the problem of immune deficiency.

Other cells which carry the T4 receptor

Although helper lymphocytes are the main target for HIV, a few subgroups of monocytes, macrophages and B lymphocytes carry a similar surface receptor. They too can be attacked by the virus. It is thought that certain cells within the central nervous system carry the receptor and this may account for the CNS manifestations of the disease.

HIV latching on to T₄ receptor

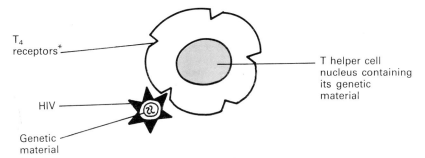

T₄ receptors*

HIV

Genetic material

T helper cell nucleus containing its genetic material

Incorporation of viral genetic material within nucleus of host cell

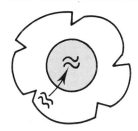

Budding and release of new virus

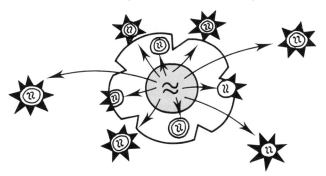

Young virus attacking other T cells

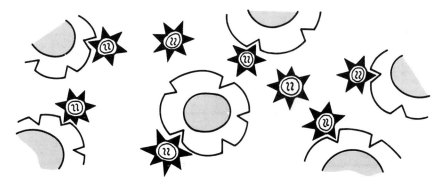

Other cells carrying T$_4$ that can be infected with HIV

- Monocytes
- Macrophages
- B lymphocytes
- Some cells within the nervous system
- Some cells within the gastrointestinal tract?
- Others?

Effects of HIV infection on the immune system

Cell-mediated immunity

Because of the interaction between HIV and T4 helper cells, it is not surprising that the cellular limb of the immune response is the one most severely affected. Classically the absolute number of helper T cells is reduced. This generally has the effect of lowering the total lymphocyte count in the AIDS patient, although this is not invariably so. The remaining infected T4 cells which have survived show evidence of impaired function. Sometimes, patients with AIDS who have clear evidence of CMI deficiency have normal numbers of helper lymphocytes. Functionally, however, a large number of these are likely to be abnormal, resulting in secondary infections and tumours. Lymphocyte response to T cell mitogens (e.g. phytohaemagglutinin) are markedly depressed in AIDS patients, as are skin tests for delayed hypersensitivity.

The suppressor and cytotoxic lymphocyte subpopulations, however, are usually normal. In the early stages, absolute levels can even be increased, presumably as a result of stimulation due to opportunistic infections, although in the terminal stages of the disease levels may fall. Because of the loss of the 'switching on' effect of T lymphocytes, the cytotoxic lymphocytes may not be very effective in spite of normal numbers. Cytotoxic and suppressor lymphocytes both contain a receptor known as T8★ and are therefore sometimes known as T8 lymphocytes. HIV, however, ignores this receptor and does not infect these cells.

Humoral immunity

In AIDS there is an increase in immunoglobulin levels, suggesting that B lymphocytes are not directly involved with the virus. This increase involves all immunoglobulin classes and is not fully understood. There is some evidence, however, that some *products* of the virus are capable of *stimulating* B cells. However, in spite of high immunoglobulin levels, the patient is unable to produce antibody to *neoantigens* (i.e. antigens to which the patient has had no prior exposure). Antibody tests in AIDS patients should not be relied upon as a diagnostic tool for the diagnosis of secondary bacterial, viral and parasitic infections.

Normal serum IgG is made up of four *subclasses*: IgG1, IgG2, IgG3, and IgG4. Recently it has been shown that the raised total IgG levels in AIDS patients are due mainly to an increase in IgG1 and IgG3 subclasses. IgG2 and IgG4 may be *subnormal*. Therefore, these patients do in fact have defects in humoral immunity in spite of having high immunoglobulin levels.

Sometimes autoantibody levels are also increased and circulating immune complexes are sometimes detected. This probably reflects the general increase in antibody production.

Non-specific immunity

Monocytes and macrophages and natural killer cell function is reduced in AIDS, contributing to the particular susceptibility to intracellular pathogens.

Immunological investigations used in the assessment of a patient who is infected with HIV

Present knowledge suggests that once HIV gains access, the individual remains infected by it for the rest of his life and so is able to pass on the virus to others. Antibody to HIV in a patient's serum does not appear to be protective but is a useful marker

---

★Now more commonly known as CD8 receptor.

to determine whether infection has occurred.

Although by far the large majority of patients infected with HIV have detectable serum antibody levels, occasionally it cannot be detected in patients from whom the virus itself has been isolated. Three groups of patients who may be antibody-negative have been recognized:

1. *Early in infection.* As with most other types of infection, it takes time for the immune system to respond. If serum is tested immediately after the individual has encountered the virus and before the immune response has been brought into play, the patient and doctor could be falsely reassured by normal antibody levels. However, a repeat test in a few weeks' time would almost invariably be positive.
2. *Late in infection.* In the last stages of frank AIDS, HIV antibody may be undetectable, reflecting a general decrease in humoral immunity.
3. *Patients unable to mount an HIV antibody response.* A small group of patients seem to be unable to mount an antibody response to HIV. They may be symptomatic or asymptomatic. Viral isolation in these patients has confirmed that infection has occurred.

Antigen or virus detection

Detection of the virus or viral antigens in the serum is more difficult than antibody testing. The virus is present in very small quantities in the blood and various tests for its presence are prolonged, time-consuming and therefore expensive. They are performed for research purposes rather than as a routine diagnostic test.

Other immunological investigations

Generalized lymphopenia, reduced numbers of T helper cells, and a general increase in immunoglobulins are usually found in the HIV-infected patient who has developed symptoms of systemic disease, opportunistic infections or tumours. They are sometimes also abnormal in the asymptomatic carrier. They are not, however, diagnostic tests and should not be used as such. However, they are likely to give important epidemiological information and guide the clinician regarding the patient's expected prognosis and how closely he should be followed up. It is likely they will be important parameters when antiviral treatment regimes become established and will indicate the patient's response to therapy.

Changes in CMI during the course of HIV infection

- Lymphopenia
- Depressed delayed hypersensitivity skin tests
- Absolute numbers of T_4 helper lymphocytes reduced
- T_8 suppressor lymphocytes may be increased
- *In vitro* activity in lymphocyte cultures depressed

Changes in humoral immunity during the course of HIV infection

- High immunoglobulin levels
- Poor response to newly encountered antigens
- IgG subclass imbalance—may be IgG2 and IgG4 deficiency
- Increase in autoantibodies
- Increase in immune complexes

> To date, AIDS, if accurately diagnosed using the proper criteria, is
>
> ALWAYS FATAL

23. Clinical features of AIDS

Once a patient infected with HIV experiences one or more of the infections or tumours at present necessary for the diagnosis of AIDS, the course of the illness is usually fairly rapidly downhill, although there will be times of apparent improvement which may make the patient feel he is on the road to recovery. At the time of writing, however, once an accurate diagnosis of AIDS is made, the disease is always eventually fatal.

Clinically, any system of the body can be involved. Patients generally first present with disease of the upper respiratory or gastrointestinal tract. Very often several conditions may coexist; for example, a patient with pneumocystis pneumonia may also have a lung infection with atypical mycobacteria and oral candidiasis. It must always be remembered that since AIDS is uniformly fatal, emphasis should always be placed on patient comfort and quality of life. Attempts to prolong life with various treatment regimens have so far been largely unsuccessful.

It is convenient to separate the physical conditions seen in the AIDS patient into four groups:

A. Infections.
B. Tumours.
C. Conditions associated with HIV infection itself.
D. Miscellaneous clinical associations.

Some of the conditions commonly seen in AIDS patients will be considered further. Those which feature as part of the current diagnostic criteria for AIDS are indicated on p. 116. The others commonly occur in AIDS patients but are also seen in the earlier stages of HIV infection.

As well as the problems associated with immuno-deficiency, there are of course immense social and emotional problems associated with the disease. These are not dealt with here but are every bit as important as the medical aspects.

Infections

Pneumocystis carinii pneumonia

Pneumonia due to this parasite is the first presenting illness in about 50% of all patients with AIDS. The average survival period, even if the patient recovers from the initial episode, is about nine months. All patients are dead within two years of their first symptoms of this infection.

Presentation is usually with gradually increasing fatigue, weight loss and fever, followed by an unproductive cough and breathlessness.

There is no evidence of person to person contact in this disease. Since a very high proportion of the normal population demonstrate antibodies to the parasite, it is thought that it normally lies dormant and it is only the severe cell-mediated depression seen in these patients that leads to its reactivation.

Mycobacterial infections

Mycobacterium tuberculosis

Infection with *Mycobacterium tuberculosis* occurs in the HIV-infected patient, affecting the bowel, lungs, or disseminated throughout the body. Because of the generalized depression in cell-mediated immunity, the Mantoux skin test may be negative in spite of fulminating infection. When positive this test is helpful diagnostically, and it indicates a better prognosis since significant T cell function is still present.

Atypical mycobacteria

Infection with the atypical *Mycobacterium avium intracellulare* is very common in the U.S.A. but not yet so in Britain. This is an environmental mycobacterium which only very rarely infects normal individuals. Unlike *M. tuberculosis*, infection with this organism signifies extensive impairment of CMI and hence generally occurs late on in the course of AIDS. Usually infection is widely disseminated throughout the body. There are no clear guidelines for treatment of this condition.

Interestingly, the classical appearance of granuloma formation and cavitation normally associated with mycobacterial infection is generally absent in AIDS patients, because these pathological processes require intact cell-mediated immunity.

Cryptosporidium

Bowel infection with this parasite existed but was not often diagnosed in patients prior to 1981. Because AIDS patients suffer a severe diarrhoeal illness due to infection with cryptosporidium the condition is being increasingly recognized in normal individuals. When the immune system is intact, it produces unpleasant but self-limiting symptoms with no long-term sequelae.

In the immune-deficient patient large volumes of watery diarrhoea are produced daily. This is associated with abdominal cramps and fever. Dehydration, malabsorption and weight loss follow and the patient can be extremely miserable because symptoms continue relentlessly.

There is at present no satisfactory treatment for cryptosporidium in the immunosuppressed patient. Fluid replacement and supportive care is all that can be offered. Temporary remissions may occur but the parasite is continually excreted until relapse occurs. Effective treatment for this miserable condition is urgently needed.

Cytomegalovirus (CMV) infections

True CMV infection is undoubtedly very common in AIDS patients. However, since nearly all homosexual men and many heterosexual adults carry the virus at some time or another, it is difficult to know whether its presence signifies infection or colonization. When true infection does occur, it is thought to be the result of viral reactivation in the immune-deficient host.

The full-blown infection results in pyrexia associated with a rash. Lungs, gastrointestinal tract, brain, meninges, and eyes may be involved. A depressed white count and thrombocytopenia are often seen. Necrosis of the bowel wall with perforation is a major complication which is often immediately fatal.

Antiviral therapy for disseminated CMV is at present under trial and the results look promising.

Epstein-Barr virus (EBV)

EBV is more commonly associated with the illness infectious mononucleosis or glandular fever. In *some*

HIV-positive patients EBV may be responsible for the lymphadenopathy syndrome frequently seen.

The virus is commonly isolated from patients with AIDS and is now thought to be responsible for a recently described condition known as '*hairy leukoplakia*' seen in these patients and those with PGL.

This condition very much resembles the white plaque of 'thrush' infection due to the yeast *Candida albicans*. The plaque, however, is not easily removed as it is in thrush, and EBV, not candida, is isolated from the lesion. Sometimes, the lesions (again like thrush) can spread into the oesophagus and result in unpleasant retrosternal discomfort, particularly when swallowing.

There is no known therapy for this condition but it may be a transient phenomenon. There is also a possibility that in the long term the lesions may go on to tumour formation.

Cryptococcal meningitis

The 'yeast-like' organism *Cryptococcus neoformans* may produce a rare form of meningitis. When seen it is usually indicative of an immunological deficiency, so, not surprisingly it is becoming an important cause of meningitis in the AIDS population.

Presentation is quite different from the acute presentation of viral or bacterial meningitis. Onset is likely to be much slower and clinical signs may be few. Examination of the cerebrospinal fluid may demonstrate few abnormal parameters. The clinician therefore must have a high awareness of the condition in these patients.

Toxoplasmosis

Central nervous system infection with the organism *Toxoplasma gondii* occurs in about 1 in 10 AIDS patients. It presents with fever, headache and focal neurological signs. The condition is generally diagnosed by computerized tomography. Other methods of diagnosis, such as serology, are not reliable. If the patient improves following a therapeutic trial of sulphadiazine and pyrimethamine, this helps confirm the diagnosis.

Progressive multifocal leucoencephalopathy

This is a condition caused by a virus (papovavirus) which leads to a progressive destruction of the white matter in the brain of an immunosuppressed individual. Diagnosis is by brain biopsy and as yet no treatment has been shown to be effective in the AIDS patient.

Recurrent salmonella bacteraemia

Gastrointestinal infection and a low-grade bacter-aemia with salmonella (particularly *Salmonella typhi-murium*) is being seen increasingly in AIDS patients. Normal regimes used to eradicate this organism in the immunocompetent host have not been effective and in the AIDS patient the condition frequently proves fatal.

Herpes simplex virus infection

A high proportion of the 'normal' population suffer intermittently from 'cold sores' which appear when the patient is temporarily 'run down', for example following a respiratory infection.

In the AIDS patient ulcers due to herpes simplex can become extensive, painful and difficult to heal. They occur on the lips and genitalia and in the homosexual patient perianally. Such lesions are extremely painful but fortunately treatment with the antiviral agent acyclovir leads to rapid improvement.

Herpes zoster

The virus responsible for herpes zoster (shingles) is the same as that responsible for chickenpox. Shingles has long been known to appear during times of temporary immunosuppression in the normal individual. In these circumstances, one dermatome only is affected. In the severely immunocompromised patient, however, herpes zoster may affect more than one dermatome or be widely disseminated. Such dissemination is associated with severe systemic disease and may prove fatal. It is important therefore that an HIV-positive patient presenting with herpes zoster is given acyclovir in an attempt to prevent dissemination.

Candidiasis

In a normal population infection with the yeast *Candida albicans* is not uncommonly seen as a complication of antibiotic therapy, because of alter-ations in the normal flora.

In the HIV-positive patient it is often one of the earliest opportunistic pathogens to be seen and may herald the onset of progression of the disease. In the early stages, the mouth only may be affected but as immunosuppression progresses lesions may spread into the oesophagus, causing difficulty swallowing. Candida septicaemia and pneumonia are seen in the terminal stages of the disease.

Tumours

Kaposi's sarcoma

Prior to 1981 Kaposi's sarcoma was a rare tumour largely confined to the Central African population. Its appearance at the onset of the AIDS epidemic in young men in the USA immediately alerted phys-icians that something very unusual was taking place. It is predominantly a tumour of the homosexual or bisexual AIDS patient, being much less frequently seen in other at-risk groups.

The skin lesions are clearly identified as reddish-purple painless papules which enlarge and eventually coalesce. Lesions involving the mucous membranes may occur, as may visceral lesions, e.g. lungs, gastrointestinal tract.

Although Kaposi's sarcoma carries with it a better prognosis than some of the opportunistic infections, treatment is not curative and it is ultimately fatal.

Non-Hodgkin's lymphoma

These tumours of B cell origin are highly malignant and difficult to treat, and occur in about 5% of the AIDS population. They not uncommonly affect the central nervous system.

Conditions associated with HIV infection itself

AIDS dementia complex

See p. 115.

Primary bowel enteropathy

Although opportunistic bowel infection is extremely common in all patients with AIDS, it has been tentatively suggested that there is another condition independent of secondary infection, where certain cells of the bowel are infected by HIV itself, leading to diarrhoea, malabsorption, and weight loss. Such symptoms are also seen in patients who have not yet been categorized as suffering from AIDS. If such direct infection of the gut does indeed take place, it is likely that the cells involved carry the T4 receptor.

Miscellaneous clinical associations

Skin conditions

Many common skin infections are frequently seen in the HIV-positive patient. As well as candida, herpes simplex and herpes zoster, other viruses, fungi and some bacteria grow unchallenged in the absence of normal cell-mediated immunity. Hence conditions such as tenia pedis, warts, molluscum contagiosum and impetigo are commonly seen. Serious bacterial infections, however, are fortunately rare, reflecting the relative unimportance of cell-mediated immune mechanisms in protection against these organisms.

A high proportion of patients with AIDS develop very dry skin. The cause is unknown but may be related to malabsorption of fatty acids due to intestinal disease.

Other conditions such as eczema, urticaria and drug hypersensitivity are common, and seem to be unrelated to infection. Their appearance probably reflects an imbalance between the various regulatory mechanisms of the immune system.

Thrombocytopenic purpura

Marked lowering of the platelet count is sometimes seen in the AIDS patient, and in the earlier stages of the disease it is often associated with PGL. Bruising, petechiae, and minor bleeding episodes are frequent but, fortunately, life-threatening bleeding has not so far been a major problem.

24. AIDS—infection control in the hospital environment

Over the years most nursing and medical staff have become very aware of the infection control issues surrounding the spread of hepatitis B. Fortunately, the risk of staff or patients accidentally contracting HIV is much less likely than the risk of contracting hepatitis B. HIV is a fragile virus which does not survive well outside body fluids and is easily destroyed. Current infection control procedures aimed at hepatitis B are therefore more than adequate to prevent the spread of HIV. Worldwide, the number of cases of accidental hospital-acquired infection is still extremely small. This, however, should not lead to complacency among hospital staff, since there are some situations which are potentially dangerous to nursing, laboratory, ancillary and medical staff.

Potentially hazardous situations

Needle stick injuries

Needle stick injuries are relatively common within a hospital population. Inadequate disposal of needles in plastic bags, for example, frequently leads to a hospital porter or domestic staff injuring themselves when lifting the bag to dispose of it. It is not unheard of for laundry staff to prick themselves on a needle left 'unattended' amongst a patient's bedding.

It has been shown that many cases of needle stick injuries occur after attempting to resheath a needle following venepuncture or intramuscular injection. Needles, therefore, should *never* be resheathed but should BE IMMEDIATELY PLACED IN A ROBUST DISPOSABLE SHARPS CONTAINER. Such containers are not without hazard. Some, for example, are poorly designed and a hospital's Control of Infection Committee should always decide which type should be used. Safety should never be compromised by using a less expensive and perhaps dangerous design of container. Even when adequate containers *are* used, human nature being what it is, no one likes to acknowledge when the sharps container is full if this involves going to a cupboard for a fresh one. So, daily, up and down the country, doctors and nurses are cramming yet another needle into containers which are already almost bulging. It then becomes difficult to put on the lid and hands are put in to remove a few needles or worse still to push them down further—sometimes pushing needles lower down through the heavy-duty cardboard. A member of staff should therefore be given responsibility to ensure that replacement empty containers are always nearby and that when the one currently in use is filled it is promptly removed.

Open skin lesions

Open skin lesions, such as cuts, abrasions, eczema, burns and impetigo, are potentially hazardous. Small such lesions should be completely covered with waterproof dressings. Widespread lesions on the hands necessitate the use of disposable gloves. No member of staff should allow broken skin to come into contact with blood or secretions from any patient, whether known to be HIV-positive or not.

Blood and body fluids

There are times in medicine and surgery when contamination with blood and other body fluids is particularly likely. Such procedures should if possible be anticipated and adequate suitable protective clothing (apron, gloves and perhaps goggles and mask) be provided for all staff involved in the procedure. Casualty presents particular problems when an extensively injured or an uncooperative patient is involved.

Patient to patient spread

This should not happen with the normal hospital practice of most civilized countries. The particular problems that have been associated with the administration of blood and blood products are dealt with later.

Decontamination, adequate sterilization procedures, use of disposable needles, syringes, catheters, etc. and a general awareness of the problem make it unlikely that patient to patient spread will occur. Many Third World countries, however, are not in such a fortunate position owing to the use of unscreened blood and recycled disposables.

AIDS has resulted in the review of many techniques in current practice and, as a result, guidelines are now widely available for most procedures involving the use of non-disposable apparatus such as fibrescopes, bronchoscopes, tonometers, etc.

Laboratory staff

As a result of present trends, HIV-positive specimens are liable to pass through any laboratory with increasing frequency. Most hospitals use 'Biohazard' or 'Danger of Infection' labels to identify known positive specimens (either hepatitis B or HIV) or high-risk specimens where serological confirmation has not been obtained. This procedure is useful in alerting laboratory staff to the potential hazard;

Some infection control procedures

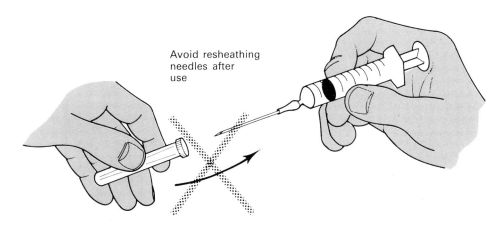

Avoid resheathing
needles after
use

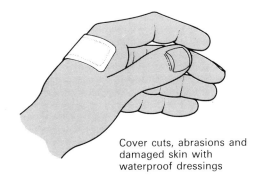

Cover cuts, abrasions and
damaged skin with
waterproof dressings

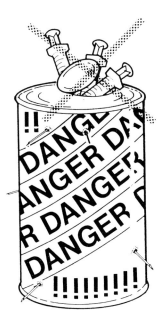

Use appropriate
container for
contaminated needles
but do not
overfill!

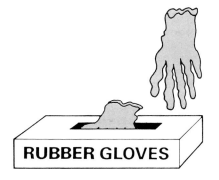

RUBBER GLOVES

Wear rubber gloves
when dealing with
body fluids

and

apron, gloves and goggles
for certain 'at-risk'
procedures

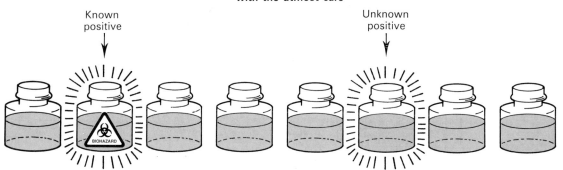

**Beware the unknown positive specimen!
ALL specimens should be handled
with the utmost care**

Known positive

Unknown positive

however, many would argue that it is the unknown specimen which creates particular problems and advocate that ALL specimens should be treated with exactly the same care as that given to one which is known to be positive.

Procedures in the laboratory follow the same principles as those in the wards. Needle prick injuries should be avoided and disposables used as far as possible. All spillages should be cleaned up immediately.

Isolation of the patient with AIDS

The fact that a patient has AIDS is *not* an indication for isolation. HIV is not transmitted by casual contact or by sharing eating utensils, etc. However, there are other reasons for isolating such patients. The newly diagnosed patient may require some time alone to come to terms with the implications of his

disease. In certain circumstances, the terminal patient retains more dignity when nursed in his or her own room. The HIV-positive patient suffering from a classical infectious disease such as tuberculosis or salmonellosis must be nursed in a single room, as must the patient who is bleeding or producing copious secretions or excretions which are not easily contained. The very immunodeficient patient sometimes requires to be given protective isolation to prevent him contracting ward pathogens which could cause him serious infectious problems.

HIV carriers among hospital staff

There is no evidence that an HIV carrier among hospital staff poses a risk to patients. Cuts and abrasions should of course be covered with a waterproof dressing and care should be taken with secretions.

Indications for isolating the HIV-positive or AIDS patient

- For psychological reasons
- The terminal patient
- Some coexisting infectious disease, e.g. salmonella, tuberculosis
- Large amounts of blood, secretions, diarrhoea
- Protective isolation for the very immunodeficient patient (neutropenia)

> It is important to be fully acquainted with local infection control policies regarding both hepatitis B virus and human immunodeficiency virus particularly in the following situations:
>
> - Skin contamination or injury
> - Gross spillage
> - Decontamination of equipment
> - Decontamination of linen
> - Decontamination of working surfaces

Accidents and spillage

Accidents unfortunately do occasionally occur and all members of staff should know the initial first aid treatment of any injury and what procedures should subseqently be followed. It is important that the hospital's occupational health physician or a senior medical physician should be involved, since immunoglobulin for hepatitis B prophylaxis may be immediately required. All cases of proven high-risk injury should be offered serial HIV antibody testing and any patient seroconverting should be recorded for epidemiological purposes.

Spillages should be dealt with immediately, using sodium hypochlorite in the recommended concentration.

Education

The importance of ongoing education cannot be over-emphasized. It should be designed to generate a feeling of involvement and lead to an understanding of why precautions are necessary. At the same time it should be emphasized that with reasonable care the risks of a member of staff contracting HIV from a patient is negligible and so patient care should in no way be compromised because of fear.

25. Prevention of community spread of HIV

Four clear facts have to be taken into account when planning measures to counteract the spread of AIDS:

1. HIV is easily transmitted by sexual contact.
2. HIV is easily spread by blood–blood contact (including secretions which contain blood).
3. HIV is frequently passed on from an infected mother to her unborn foetus.
4. HIV is NOT spread by casual everyday non-sexual contact.

Spread via sexual contact

There is no doubt that the AIDS epidemic is basically *venereal*, involving *both homosexual and heterosexual* populations. Spread via blood is secondary in the epidemic since venereal spread will have taken place somewhere earlier in the transmission line. The *rate* of spread of the epidemic is a reflection of the involvement of large numbers of sexual partners.

Unfortunately, realization of the size of the problem was too late, since there is now a large pool of HIV-infected asymptomatic carriers in each continent who are capable of passing on the disease. The numbers in this pool are not accurately known since screening for HIV antibody status is not routinely carried out among random populations in most countries. The first stage of any prevention programme must be to educate each nation so that individuals can identify whether they are in an 'at-risk' group. Secondly, they should be given easily understood accurate information on how to modify their behaviour so that they can protect themselves and others. In most countries, pressure is not put on such at-risk individuals to have their HIV antibody status determined, because of the complicated social, ethical and psychological problems that are now well identified in those in whom the result is positive. Such an attitude will of course change if and when satisfactory treatment for the asymptomatic individual becomes available.

A very significant degree of success with such strategies has already been seen with the homosexual population. This group have taken the threat extremely seriously and most have decreased their numbers of sexual partners substantially. Many are now indeed celibate and many more are restricting sexual practices to one partner only. Whether the outcome will be similar in the highly promiscuous heterosexual group remains to be seen. It is extremely unlikely that society will see an end to prostitution, and this, 'the oldest of professions', has now become very clearly intertwined with drug addiction. This is particularly so in Scotland where Edinburgh within recent years has demonstrated an unexpected and extremely alarming rate of spread among drug addicts. In this city addicts rely very heavily on prostitution to fund their craving. It would be extremely difficult to find the large amounts of money required daily by addicts by any method other than prostitution. Since many addicts know or suspect that they have already contracted the virus they feel they have no need to protect themselves. Not infrequently they despise their 'clients' and care not in the least whether they pass on the disease to them. In the face of such a background, the problem of education becomes enormous, if not impossible.

The second stage of a prevention programme must be to educate the majority of the population who have much fewer sexual contacts than those described above to reduce the risk of their contracting the disease to virtually zero. Clearly, total lack of sexual contact is neither practical or desirable to most individuals. The safest alternative choice therefore is one of mutual trust in agreeing 'one partner for life', assuming of course that neither carries the virus at the start of the relationship. Such a practice is 100% safe, assuming that other risk-associated procedures such as needle sharing are not practised. When an individual decides that for him or her there will be several sexual partners, then a condom should always be used (and used properly) for protection. This leads to a substantial reduction in the risk of contracting AIDS.

Casual sex using condoms does not, however, decrease the risk to zero and education programmes should not omit to make this point clearly. Many individuals, given the choice between a monogamous relationship which has virtually no risk and a polygamous relationship using condoms which has low risk, may feel that any risk at all is too high for such a serious disease. It should not therefore be assumed that individuals will not change their sexual habits when education programmes are being designed. The options and risks open to them should be clearly presented with equal emphasis so that individuals are fully informed before they make their choice.

HIV *is* spread by:
- Sexual contact (homosexual and heterosexual)
- Blood to blood contact (including secretions containing blood)
- Mother to foetus

HIV is *not* spread by:
- Everyday non-sexual contact

Spread via blood and secretions

Haemophiliacs who depend on factor VIII or cryoprecipitate for maintaining haemostasis were unknowingly and tragically caught up in the AIDS epidemic. The commercial production of each vial of factor VIII contains clotting factors from literally thousands of donors. It is not surprising therefore that some of these donors were HIV-positive. Following realization that large numbers of haemophiliacs were antibody-positive, the manufacturing technique used in the production of factor VIII has been modified to involve heat treatment. It appears to prevent the problem and hopefully no more new haemophiliacs will be infected.

The risk of acquiring HIV via transfused blood or plasma in the Western world is now extremely unlikely. Nowadays, in most countries blood is screened for evidence of HIV infection before it is given to the patient. This risk is now minimal, although theoretically an occasional HIV carrier could be missed who is antibody-negative. Suitably designed questionnaires are used to help exclude the 'at risk' donor.

A much greater problem that has emerged is the rapid spread of the virus in some areas among the drug addict population, due largely to the sharing of needles and syringes. Clearly the ideal situation is to stop drug addiction at every step. No effort should be spared to prevent young people from starting the habit, both by education and the effective control of drug trafficking. This ideal, however, is difficult to achieve and time has already run out in some areas. Education of drug addicts themselves will not be effective quickly enough, if at all, and so the decision facing governments is whether to take the ethically difficult step to provide sterile needles and syringes and perhaps the drugs themselves to the addict population. Preliminary trials along these lines have been initiated in some countries, including Britain. They will require to be shown to be effective in their eventual outcome, otherwise all that will have been achieved is an apparent 'condoning' of drug abuse.

Materno-foetal spread

A new wave of tragic consequences of the AIDS epidemic has now emerged. HIV-infected mothers are capable of passing the infection to their unborn children. The chances of this happening are not absolutely clear, but it is likely that more than 50% of infants born to such mothers will be infected. What proportion of these children will go on to develop AIDS is not yet known.

The background of the mothers involved varies. The majority are drug addicts, but some have acquired their infection heterosexually and others by receiving a blood transfusion. There have also been cases of infection occurring as the result of artificial insemination from an infected semen donor. There may also be a degree of risk of spread from colostrum and milk, but this risk has not been quantified.

It should be remembered that the results of a positive HIV antibody test in a child born to an infected mother may be difficult to interpret. Maternal IgG which has crossed the placenta will result in a positive test in the child during the first few months of life. If this persists beyond four months it reflects genuine infection in the child.

At the present time, all HIV-infected women are advised not to become pregnant. If already pregnant the mother should be asked to consider termination.

A baby born to an infected mother should in civilized countries *not* be breast fed. In the meantime, however, advice to infected mothers in the Third World *should* be to breast feed since the risks of contracting other infections by not doing so may be greater to the baby than the risk of contracting HIV infection.

Other possible means of spread

There are other procedures which involve risks to a varying degree. These involve blood–blood contact but have not been included above.

Tissue transplantation

Organ transplant cards are widely carried and some patients may already have them on their person at the time of a fatal accident. It is important that education programmes emphasize that at-risk individuals should not only withdraw from voluntary blood donation but should also destroy organ donor cards, should not donate semen, and should not leave their bodies for undesignated 'research'.

Commercial procedures without medical surveillance

Spread via 'sharps' in the form of ear-piercing, tattooing, acupuncture and shaving can theoretically take place. Unfortunately, one can never be sure that infection control procedures are adequately carried out or that disposables are being used. Although the risk may be very small it must nonetheless be there and this point should clearly be made as part of the general education programme against AIDS.

Procedures within the home

Most people regard their homes as havens of safety. While sharing cooking utensils, cutlery, crockery, etc. is considered safe, HIV potentially could be passed on via shared toothbrushes, razors, and perhaps even scissors and hairbrushes if a member of the family who is a carrier has broken skin.

It is worthwhile to emphasize that it is good hygienic practice that each member of a household should have his or her own personal items and they should not be used by anyone else.

Vaccination

Obviously this is an area into which is being put a great deal of money and effort. Many hurdles have to be crossed before protection from AIDS by vaccination becomes a reality. Until that time comes, and it is probably several years away, individuals must rely on changing their behaviour patterns in order to protect themselves.

26. The management of the HIV-infected patient
Counselling

Management of the potentially HIV-infected individual really starts before the serum is taken for antibody testing. At this stage the patient is extremely anxious but has not fully thought through the implications if the result of the test proves to be positive. Professional counselling is extremely important at this stage *before* the patient takes the decision to have the investigation performed. Indeed, he may decide *not* to take the test, in which case as an individual at risk he should be counselled further regarding the subsequent protection of himself and others.

Immediate and ongoing counselling is of course equally important in the patient whose antibody test is positive. Further discussion of this aspect is, however, outside the scope of this book.

The adoption of strategies that may prevent progression of the disease

Some individuals may argue that once it has been confirmed that they are HIV-positive then life may be too short for them to alter their lifestyle. In the case of the homosexually or heterosexually promiscuous, or in the drug addict, there is some evidence suggesting that exposure to unrelated new infections, e.g. gonococci, herpes viruses, staphylococci, candida, hepatitis, will precipitate or hasten the progression of the asymptomatic HIV stage or PGL to the full-blown AIDS syndrome. The concept that the patient can possibly have a degree of control over his future should therefore be introduced early.

Immunologically, the reason behind such a theory would be as follows:

1. On initial HIV infection, virus is incorporated into a small number of T helper cells. The numbers involved are too small to have an effect on CMI and the patient remains asymptomatic.

2. The virus remains inaccessible and inactive within the cells for a variable length of time, awaiting a situation that will activate helper cells and prepare them for cell division.

3. Any type of infection will normally 'switch on' the immune system, including T4 helper lymphocytes.

4. This activation will simultaneously 'switch on' viral replication.

5. Young virus will then be released into the circulation. They will seek out more T4 receptors on as yet unaffected helper lymphocytes, infect them and the cycle will repeat itself until most helper cells are infected or killed by the virus. Increasing lymphocyte destruction will be manifest by progressive immunodeficiency leading eventually to frank AIDS.

It seems reasonable then, until more is known about the factors precipitating AIDS, to advise *all* patients to minimize their risks of infection if this is at all possible.

Pregnancy can also be regarded as an antigenic stimulus which may activate T4 lymphocytes. The foetus is after all 50% paternal, i.e. it is recognized as foreign to the mother. Mechanisms must clearly come into play in the normal pregnancy to prevent foetal rejection; however, it is likely that a degree of immunological stimulation continually takes place.

Not only does the HIV-positive mother carry the burden that she may produce an infected infant, time and again it has been shown also that her own health is likely to deteriorate with the clinical features of a full-blown AIDS syndrome manifesting themselves. Clear guidelines should therefore be given to all female patients to avoid pregnancy, although of course the ultimate decision must rest with the patient.

In view of the above, it seems sensible that HIV-infected patients should not only *avoid* precipitating factors but should adopt a lifestyle which keeps them as nutritionally fit as possible. No protein, vitamin or mineral deficiencies should be allowed to develop and crash diets should be avoided. Many may have

---

A positive HIV test is not a death sentence!
The evidence so far suggests that the HIV-infected patient should take particular care of all aspects of his health. This may avoid or slow progression to AIDS

slipped into the 'junk food' routine and ongoing support by a dietitian may be very helpful.

Some patients may already be receiving immuno-suppressive agents for entirely unrelated conditions, e.g. systemic steroids for asthma or serious skin conditions. Such therapy is potentially dangerous in these patients and should be discontinued unless the condition being treated is in itself life-threatening.

Secondary infection and tumours

Once the patient becomes classified within group IV and secondary infections and tumours make their appearance, therapy has to be directed towards their treatment and the patient hospitalized if this is required. Psychological support at this stage is also extremely important because the patient is invariably very aware of the ominous significance of his symptoms.

Antiviral agents

Several antiviral agents are at present on clinical trial throughout the world, mainly in established AIDS patients. It is too early yet to be optimistic and effects so far demonstrated are minimal. There are many problems associated with antiviral therapy for this condition and it is likely that we are several years away from effective therapy.

Immunopotentiation

Theoretically, it might be possible to help reconstitute the damaged immune system by the adminis-tration of substances produced normally by the cells which have been destroyed by this condition. Alternatively, bone marrow transplantation may be expected to restore the immune system in a way similar to that seen in the treatment of leukaemia or some of the serious congenital immunodeficiency syndromes.

So far no major advances have been made in this area but techniques may improve and ultimately patients may benefit.

Conclusion

Although at the moment the overall problems surrounding the AIDS epidemic appear to be over-whelming and depressing, it should be remembered that large advances have been made regarding the aetiology, epidemiology and understanding of the disease mechanisms in a very short time. Much time, money, and effort is being expended world-wide and doors of international communication for the transfer of information are wide open. There is no reason why we should not see very significant advances, with the possibility of vaccination, antiviral therapy or immunorestoration within the next dec-ade. This at least gives those already infected something to hold on to.

Control of the epidemic today, however, depends on individuals, not scientists. Each one of us as never before must take responsibility for our own health and behavioural patterns. We are already committed to leaving a legacy of fear and disease to the generations that follow. Let that legacy be as small as possible!

Section D

Immunological investigation and procedures

The investigation of a patient suspected of having an immunological problem

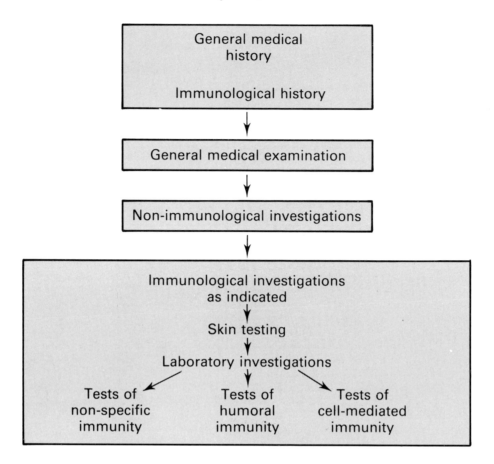

27. Introduction

The investigation of a patient suspected of having an immunological problem

Many immunological conditions such as those associated with severe recurrent infections are extremely rare. It is important, therefore, that commoner causes of such symptoms be excluded before embarking on a full immunological investigation. It would be unreasonable, for example, to investigate cell-mediated immunity or polymorph function in a patient suffering from recurrent infections before excluding diabetes mellitus—a condition well known to be associated with infective problems.

It is also worth remembering that many tests of immune function are expensive, time-consuming and require considerable technical expertise. Some-

times the results can be difficult to evaluate.

Some immunological investigations are essential for the accurate diagnosis of immunological conditions; some are helpful, whereas others are of academic interest only and contribute very little to patient management.

Where expensive and time-consuming investigations are being considered, a clinical immunologist should be contacted both to discuss the usefulness of the proposed investigations and to give the laboratory due warning so that prior preparations can be made.

Immunological history

A.	History of infections

B.	History of allergies

C.	Vaccination history

D.	History of possible autoimmune symptoms

E.	Drug history

F.	Family history

History

Immunological history

As in any other branch of medicine or surgery, clinical investigation begins at the bedside by talking to the patient. This takes the form of a detailed medical history, but in assessing immunological status certain questions should be asked.

History of infections

Are recurrent infections of recent onset or have they been present since early childhood?

What is the site of infection?

What is the organism involved? (Remember that bacterial infections suggest a defect of humoral immunity, viral and fungal infections and tuberculosis are associated with cell-mediated defects, and that where unusual organisms of low virulence are implicated, an immunological abnormality is likely.)

History of allergies

Is there a history of asthma, eczema, hay fever, or urticaria? If so do any obvious allergens precipitate these symptoms? Are symptoms seasonal suggesting pollen allergy? Is there a history of diarrhoea following ingestion of certain foods suggesting food allergy?

Is there any history of contact dermatitis suggesting allergy to substances such as nickel or plants such as primula?

Is there any history of a reaction to bee or wasp stings or insect bites?

Vaccination history

Has there been any unusually severe reaction to some vaccines?

Have vaccines apparently resulted in the immunity intended?

History of possible autoimmune disease

Is there a history of joint symptoms, anaemia, haematuria, or any other vague systemic upset?

Drug history

Is the patient receiving any drugs such as steroids that are capable of suppressing the immune system?

Immunological investigations

In vivo tests

Skin tests for delayed
hypersensitivity

Skin tests for immediate
hypersensitivity

Provocation tests

In vitro tests

Tests of non-specific immunity	Tests of humoral immunity	Tests of cell-mediated immunity
Differential white cell count Erythrocyte sedimentation rate Complement activity Neutrophil function tests Measurement of C-reactive protein	Immunoglobulin IgG, IgA and IgM quantitation IgE estimation Immunoelectrophoresis Cryoglobulin detection Specific antibody production Circulating immune complex detection	T and B cell quantitation Lymphocyte cultures

Family history

Is there a family history of autoimmune disease, allergy, or other immunological disorders?

Is there any history of sudden infant deaths, raising the possibility of a severe inherited immune deficiency?

General medical examination

A thorough medical examination may reveal signs of immunological disease. However, it is important to look for signs of non-immunological disease accounting for the patient's symptoms. For example, finger clubbing with signs of respiratory disease may signify congenital heart disease rather than a primary immunodeficiency.

Non-immunological investigations

Following history taking and examination, non-immunological investigations such as urinalysis, full blood count, differential white cell count, ESR (erythrocyte sedimentation rate), chest X-ray, urea and electrolytes, and liver function tests should be performed. These may sometimes point to an immunological abnormality.

Immunological investigations

Before embarking on immunological investigation one should consider carefully which investigations are likely to be helpful in a given clinical situation. It is impossible in practice to screen all limbs of the immune response in every patient vaguely suspected of having an immunological disorder. Some investigations such as immunoglobulin estimation and immunoelectrophoresis can be done routinely without prior arrangement with the laboratory. However, other investigations such as lymphocyte cultures and chemotactic assays are time-consuming and require planning. Hence they can only be performed following prior consultation with laboratory staff.

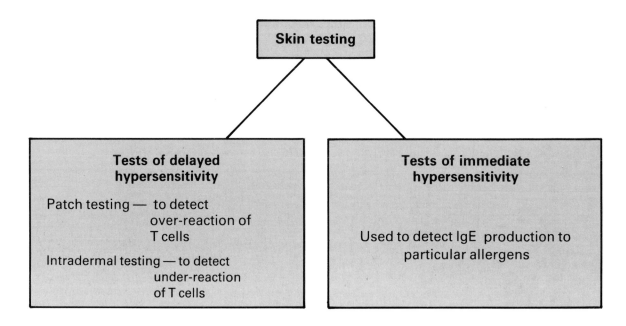

28. *In vivo* tests

Skin testing

Three types of skin testing are commonly performed and each type gives entirely different information about the patient:

1. The *patch test* gives information about *hypersensitivity* of the *cell-mediated system*.
2. *Intradermal skin testing for delayed hypersensitivity* detects possible *underactivity* of the *cell-mediated system*.
3. *Prick testing* for *immediate hypersensitivity* gives information regarding the *IgE antibody system*.

The antigens chosen for each type of skin test are totally different.

Other *in vivo* techniques such as the *Rebuck skin window* are not usually employed on a routine basis.

Although the techniques are simple to perform, the interpretation of results can be difficult, and it is recommended that these tests are performed only at clinics where the physician has experience in the interpretation of large numbers of positive and negative results.

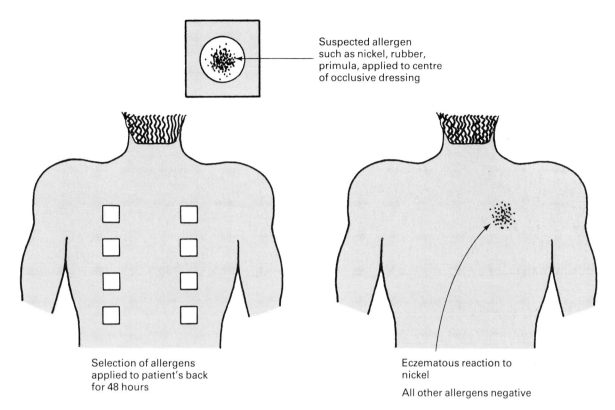

The patch test

Suspected allergen such as nickel, rubber, primula, applied to centre of occlusive dressing

Selection of allergens applied to patient's back for 48 hours

Eczematous reaction to nickel

All other allergens negative

Patch testing

This test is made use of mainly by dermatologists in the diagnosis of *contact dermatitis*. It involves applying a small amount of the suspected contact allergen to the skin of the back under an occlusive dressing. This is kept in place for a period of 48 hours. A small patch of eczema developing at the site of allergen in question constitutes a positive result and the patient can then be advised to avoid the offending agent if this is possible. False-positive patch tests are not uncommon in patients with der-matitis, and patients receiving corticosteroid therapy frequently demonstrate false-negative results.

Weakly positive patch test results should always be interpreted with caution. It should be remembered that, once a substance has been implicated as damaging to the patient, his lifestyle may have to be radically altered in order to avoid the offending substance. In some cases this may mean a change of occupation with loss of income.

Intradermal skin testing for anergy

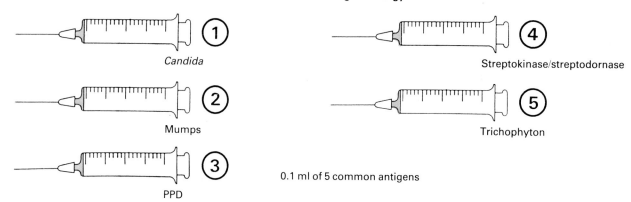

① Candida

② Mumps

③ PPD

④ Streptokinase/streptodornase

⑤ Trichophyton

0.1 ml of 5 common antigens

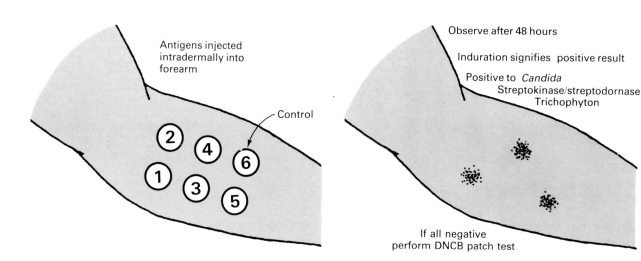

Antigens injected intradermally into forearm

Control

Observe after 48 hours

Induration signifies positive result

Positive to Candida
Streptokinase/streptodornase
Trichophyton

If all negative
perform DNCB patch test

Delayed hypersensitivity skin tests for anergy

Anergy, or a state of cell-mediated unresponsiveness can be implied if a patient fails to show a response to any of a battery of common antigens to which he has been exposed at some time in the past.

In Britain one can generally assume that an individual's immune system has previously encountered one or more of the following antigens due to previous exposure to various microorganisms:

Candida
Mumps
Purified protein derivative (PPD) (from the tubercle bacillus)
Streptokinase/streptodornase (from the streptococcus)
Trichophyton

The skin testing technique involves injecting 0.1 ml of each extract intradermally into the forearm and observing it over a period of 48 hours. After this period a positive reactor demonstrates induration and erythema at the site of the injection. If there is no reaction to any of the five antigens then the patient *may* have deficient cell-mediated immunity. This can be confirmed by attempting to sensitize to *dinitrochlorobenzene* (DNCB), a potent but previously unencountered antigen. This technique involves a patch test rather than an intradermal skin test, and using this potent sensitizer about 90% of all individuals with an intact cell-mediated system will develop a local site of allergic contact dermatitis.

Skin tests for immediate hypersensitivity

Antigens dropped on to skin which is then lightly pricked

control

Wheal and flare reaction to house dust mite (HDM) and pollen after a few minutes

Skin tests for immediate hypersensitivity

These skin tests are used to identify which patients are capable of producing IgE antibody to various antigens. They are therefore used in the investigation of patients with *atopic eczema* or *asthma*.

The technique most commonly used is the *prick test*. This involves placing a small amount of the antigen in question on the skin of the patient's forearm. The skin is then gently scarified very superficially. A positive result to an offending allergen is recorded if a wheal of erythema appears within 10 minutes. The reaction is over within about an hour. The time sequence is therefore entirely different from the cell-mediated reactions previously described.

Intradermal skin testing for immediate hypersensitivity can also be performed, but in general this is less satisfactory than prick testing.

The antigens chosen depend on the history of the patient. However, *house dust mite, grass pollen, cat* and *dog antigens* are generally always included. In general, skin testing shows a good correlation with history when inhaled allergens are involved. Food allergens, however, do not seem to be readily detected by the prick test.

It should always be remembered that there is a small but well-recognized risk of an anaphylactic

reaction as a result of skin testing a patient who is extremely sensitive to a particular allergen. *Adrenaline* should always be at hand when these techniques are being performed. Measuring specific IgE by *in vitro* methods is safer in a patient who has a previous history of a serious hypersensitivity reaction.

Skin testing is also difficult in patients who suffer from *dermatographism*. These patients develop a wheal and flare simply on stroking the skin without contact with allergen. Sometimes also the skin may be so severely eczematous that skin testing is not practicable. In these situations *in vitro* methods of detecting IgE must be relied upon.

Provocation tests

Respiratory provocation tests can sometimes be used to determine the significance of a particular allergen, or to monitor the effects of treatment. That is, instead of presenting the allergen to the skin as previously described, it is inhaled and the effect on the respiratory tract observed.

These investigations can precipitate a severe asthmatic attack and should always be performed in hospital by an experienced physician.

★ HDM stands for 'house dust mite'.

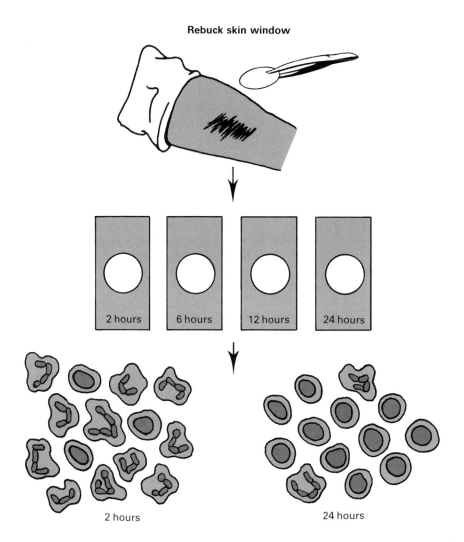

Rebuck skin window

2 hours

24 hours

Rebuck skin window

An *in vivo* assessment of non-specific immunity can be made by the *Rebuck skin window* technique. This test, however, is difficult to quantitate and can be rather impractical to perform on a young child. The test is therefore generally omitted routinely.

The test is performed by abrading the patient's forearm skin using a sterile scalpel and covering the abrasion with a sterile glass coverslip. This is then covered with a dressing and left *in situ* for a given length of time (e.g. 2 hours). In the normal individual, neutrophils will migrate to the site during this time. The coverslip is then removed and replaced by a fresh one which is left in place for a further few hours. This procedure is repeated over several hours. Each coverslip is then stained, mounted on a slide and examined under the microscope.

In the normal person the predominant cell during the first 6-hour period is the neutrophil. This cell is gradually replaced by mononuclear cells and after 24 hours these cells predominate.

<table>
<tr><td>

In vitro immunological investigations requiring prior arrangement with lab

- Neutrophil function tests
- T and B cell quantitation
- Lymphocyte culture

</td><td>

In vitro immunolgoical investigations requiring no prior arrangement

- Immunoglobulin G,A,M quantitation
- IgE estimation
- Immunoelectrophoresis
- Specific antibody detection

</td></tr>
</table>

29. *In vitro* tests

The collection of specimens

The majority of investigations in clinical immunology (e.g. immunoglobulin estimations) are performed on *serum* samples. In this case, 10 ml of clotted blood should be sent to the laboratory where the serum is separated by centrifugation and stored at $-20\,°C$ in a deep freeze until the relevant tests are performed.

There are, however, the following important exceptions.

Lymphocyte and neutrophil function tests

Blood should be collected into bottles containing *preservative free heparin* as anticoagulant.

Since these tests are performed on live cells there should be no delay in transporting the specimens to the laboratory. Blood should always be taken from a *normal control* subject at the same time and the control blood should be treated in exactly the same way as the test blood. Moreover, in children under two years of age the control blood should be from an *age-matched* donor. This is because in young children neutrophil function is less efficient and lymphocyte turnover is more rapid than it is in adults. Age-matching is less important in older children and in adults.

Secretions

In the investigation of possible IgA deficiency it is often helpful to look for the presence of secretory IgA in, for example, saliva or jejunal juice. It is advisable to seek advice from the laboratory about collection of these specimens since certain precautions must be taken to avoid proteolysis.

Urine

In the investigation of paraproteinaemias, immunoelectrophoretic studies should be performed on urine for the demonstration of Bence-Jones protein.

A suitable specimen would be 50 ml of fresh urine in a sterile container.

Cryoglobulins

Cryoglobulins are immunoglobulins which precipitate at $4\,°C$. If high levels of cryoglobulin are present in the serum, the patient may show clinical symptoms and signs due to vascular damage precipitated by cold exposure.

For the detection of cryoglobulins, it is of great importance that blood should be taken into a *warmed syringe* and held at $37\,°C$ for 2 hours while clotting.

The laboratory should be informed prior to bleeding the patient so that arrangements can be made for transporting the blood at $37\,°C$ (e.g. in a thermos flask).

Complement

Conditions of collection and storage of specimens for measurement of individual components of the complement system are critical, since *in vitro* activation of the complement cascade must be avoided. Blood should be collected into EDTA whenever possible, and plasma separated by centrifugation within 1–2 hours of collection and stored at $-70\,°C$ until testing. Repeated thawing and freezing of specimens induces complement conversion and should be avoided.

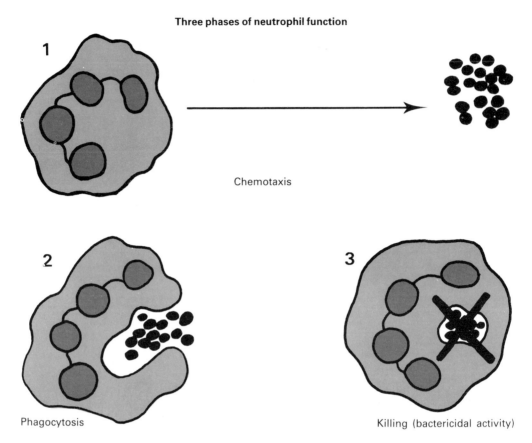

Three phases of neutrophil function

1

Chemotaxis

2

Phagocytosis

3

Killing (bactericidal activity)

A defect in any one phase may give rise to recurrent
infections

Tests of non-specific immunity
Neutrophil function

When haematologists report a *white blood count*, they estimate the *numbers* of white blood cells in a peripheral blood smear. When they report a *differential white count*, they indicate the *proportion* of white cells that make up the total white count, and when they report on a *blood film*, they comment on the *structural appearances* of the red blood cells and white blood cells.

These reports, however, give no indication of whether the white cells are capable of normal function. In theory, it is quite possible that cells may look normal and be present in normal numbers and yet be incapable of functioning efficiently.

At present, only tests of polymorph and lymphocyte function are performed routinely. Investigation into macrophage, eosinophil and basophil function is at present only performed at research level.

There are adequate *in vitro* tests to measure only some neutrophil functions, i.e. *chemotaxis, phagocytosis* and *bactericidal activities*. Normal values for neutrophil function vary between laboratories and even from day to day in the same laboratory. *It is always necessary, therefore, to compare the cells of the patient with those of the normal control tested on the same day.*

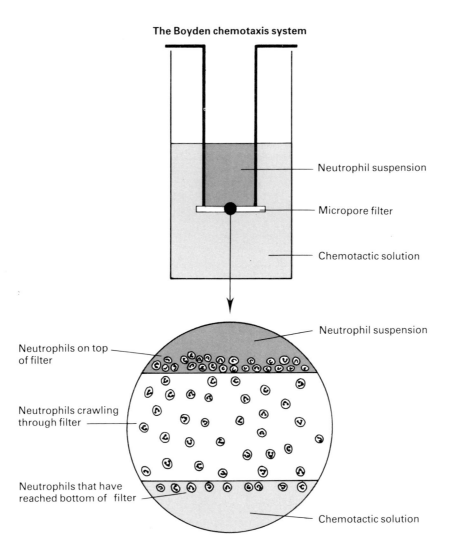

The Boyden chemotaxis system

Neutrophil suspension

Micropore filter

Chemotactic solution

Neutrophil suspension

Neutrophils on top of filter

Neutrophils crawling through filter

Neutrophils that have reached bottom of filter

Chemotactic solution

Chemotaxis

Neutrophil chemotaxis (i.e. the ability of the neutrophil to move towards a chemical attractant and hence its ability to move towards an infecting organism) is usually examined using a micropore filter technique. A chamber★ with compartments and a filter separating them is used. The patient's cells are placed in the upper compartment and a substance which attracts neutrophils (e.g. casein) is placed in the lower compartment. Such a substance is known as a *chemotactic factor*. The chemotactic factor diffuses up through the filter so forming a concentration gradient and the cells are attracted to move into the filter. The filter has pores of such a size as to allow cells to squeeze through by active locomotion, but not drop through passively.

After a period of incubation, the filter is removed, cleared and stained. The distance the neutrophils have migrated through the filter is determined using a microscope.

The patient's cells are also incubated in the absence of chemotactic substance to demonstrate random unstimulated migration.

★i.e. a *Boyden chamber*.

Polarization assay

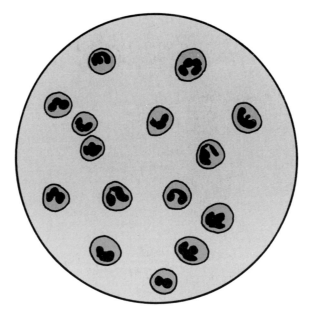

Normal
unstimulated
neutrophils

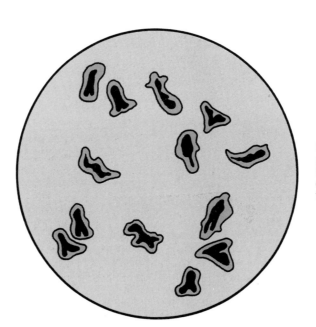

Neutrophils
polarized after
incubation with
chemotactic
factor

The results obtained using the Boyden assay can be misleading owing to the interaction of the neutrophils with the filter.

A simpler and more convenient method of assessing the chemotactic response of neutrophils is by direct observation of individual cells in a polarization assay.

Normal unstimulated neutrophils are 95% spherical in shape. In the presence of chemotactic factors, however, they acquire the shape of a migrating cell, i.e. they become *polarized*.

In a polarization assay the patient's neutrophils are incubated with a chemotactic factor and then simply fixed and examined microscopically. Any cell deviating from a spherical outline is said to be polarized.

Nitroblue tetrazolium test

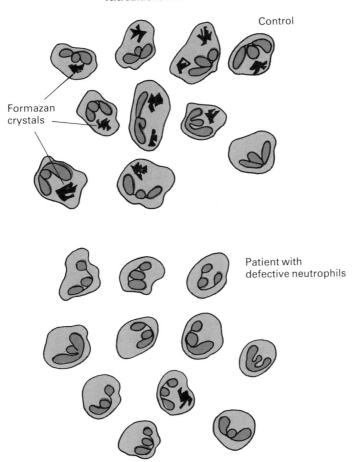

Control

Formazan
crystals

Patient with
defective neutrophils

Phagocytosis and killing

At present the *nitroblue tetrazolium (NBT) test* is used as a rapid and simple screening method for detecting gross defects of neutrophil phagocytosis and/or killing. However, it is possible that in the future the technique of *chemiluminescence* will be a more sensitive method of detecting these defects.

NBT test

Nitroblue tetrazolium (NBT) is a dye which, in the oxidized form, is soluble and has a pale yellow colour but which, when reduced, becomes blue-black and forms crystals (*formazan crystals*).

In the test, the patient's cells are exposed to the yellow NBT dye. Unstimulated neutrophils do not ingest this dye, but if the cells are stimulated to phagocytic activity by adding serum containing bacterial products like endotoxin, they ingest the dye and reduce it intracellularly. This can be easily seen under the microscope since neutrophils which have reduced NBT have blue dots of formazan in their cytoplasm. By counting 200 cells, the percentage of the patient's neutrophils containing blue deposits can be determined and compared with normal neutrophils. Only about 10% of normal unstimulated neutrophils from human blood reduce NBT. However, once stimulated in the presence of endotoxin the number of neutrophils reducing NBT rises normally to at least 80%.

The NBT test is a measure of both the phagocytic function and the bactericidal activity of neutrophils.

Chemiluminescence

The metabolic 'burst' in neutrophils which occurs during phagocytosis and killing generates light which can be measured using a luminometer. This technique is known as *chemiluminescence* and it is now being used to measure the bactericidal function of neutrophils. It is, however, an *indirect* measure and should always be correlated with *direct* assessment of phagocytosis and killing.

Visual measurement of phagocytosis

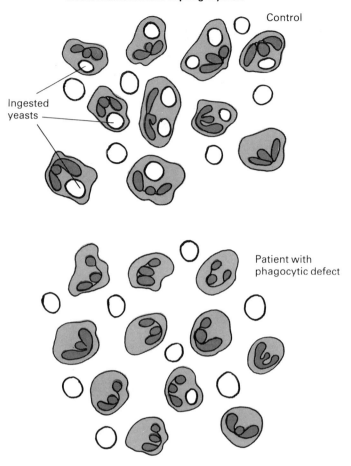

Control

Ingested
yeasts

Patient with
phagocytic defect

Phagocytosis

Most methods for measuring phagocytic function *alone* involve *direct visual counting of ingested particles* using a microscope.

The patient's neutrophils are incubated for a brief period with inert particles (e.g. heat-killed yeast) in the presence of fresh serum. Stained slide preparations are then made. Two hundred cells are examined under the microscope to determine the average number of yeasts ingested per patient's neutrophil. This can be compared with the number phagocytosed by normal cells.

An alternative method uses staphylococci. The patient's neutrophils are incubated with a fixed number of living staphylococci to allow phagocytosis to occur. The supernatant containing any residual unphagocytosed organisms is then separated by centrifugation, plated on to blood agar and incubated overnight. Counting of colonies of growth the next day gives an indication of the number of organisms *not* phagocytosed.

Opsonization

Normal serum contains substances that enhance phagocytosis; i.e. certain types of antibody and components of the complement system. These substances are called *opsonins*. Sometimes serum can be deficient in these substances. Such serum is then said to have *defective opsonizing activity*. It is possible to detect this by adding the patient's serum to a mixture of *normal control* neutrophils and yeast particles.

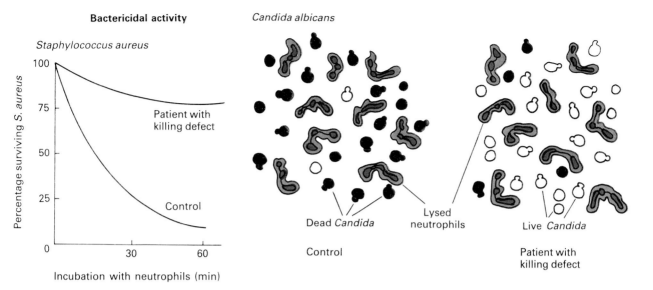

Bactericidal activity

Staphylococcus aureus

Candida albicans

Dead *Candida*

Lysed neutrophils

Live *Candida*

Control

Patient with killing defect

Killing (bactericidal activity)

The killing of organisms already ingested by neutrophils is measured by counting the numbers of organisms that can survive intracellularly after phagocytosis has taken place. Staphylococci or yeasts are commonly used in this test.

1. After incubation of the patient's cells with a suspension of staphylococci to allow phagocytosis to occur, all remaining extracellular bacteria are killed with an antibiotic solution, and incubation is continued to allow intracellular killing to take place. Finally, the patient's neutrophils are ruptured and the residual live bacteria are plated on to culture medium and counted.
2. When yeasts are used, the patient's cells are ruptured after incubation and a solution of blue dye added. Dead yeast cells take up the dye within a minute or so whereas living cells exclude it. The suspension is then examined microscopically and 200 yeast cells are counted to determine the percentage of yeasts killed.

These tests permit differentiation between phagocytic and intracellular killing defects. However, they require large volumes of blood and the culture of organisms before and after incubation with neutrophils, taking trained personnel 2–3 days to perform.

Summary

The study of neutrophil function is complex and best investigated in a specialized laboratory. The indications for investigating patients for defective neutrophil function are recurrent severe or chronic infections often with unusual organisms. Often there is a family history of similar problems. The patient's humoral immune state should first have been investigated before embarking on neutrophil function tests, since hypogammaglobulinaemia is a commoner and more readily recognizable cause of immunodeficiency.

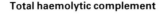

Total haemolytic complement

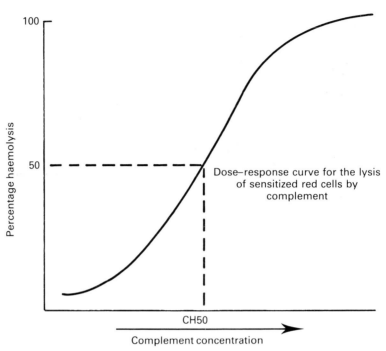

Dose–response curve for the lysis of sensitized red cells by complement

Laboratory investigation of the complement system

Complement levels are elevated in most inflammatory diseases. A laboratory finding of raised levels therefore offers little information to the clinician. Low levels, however, are found in some important medical conditions. Investigation of the complement system is therefore indicated:

1. In conditions in which a genetic defect is suspected, e.g. patients presenting with recurrent infections or with the rare condition of hereditary angioneurotic oedema where there is a deficiency of one of the regulator enzymes and the complement sequence activates in an uncontrolled manner.
2. In the assessment of patients suffering from conditions where complement consumption is playing a part in the disease process, e.g. systemic lupus erythematosus, some forms of glomerulonephritis and other varieties of immune complex disorders.

Two main types of test are frequently performed for the assessment of complement activity:

1. *Functional complement assays*
2. *Quantitation of individual components*

Functional complement assays

Total haemolytic complement is a useful screening test to demonstrate the correct functioning of the whole of the classical pathway C1–C9. The assay is based on the ability of the intact complement system to rupture sheep red blood cells coated with antibody to sheep red cells. Haemoglobin released by such cell lysis can be measured spectrophotometrically with great accuracy. Lysis of an aliquot of the red cells in distilled water gives a reading for the total releasable haemoglobin, and the ratio of one to the other indicates the percentage of cells lysed. These values, when plotted against amount of active complement, give a curve the slope of which is steepest around 50% lysis and therefore small differences in complement activity result in the greatest differences in observed lysis. For this reason results are usually expressed in *CH50 units*—one unit being the volume of patient's serum needed to lyse 50% of a standard suspension of coated red cells.

Haemolytic assays for measuring the function of the individual components of the complement system are also available, but are expensive and time-consuming. They are seldom necessary for clinical purposes other than in the detection of genetic defects where a complement component is present in normal levels but is functionally inactive.

Radial immunodiffusion

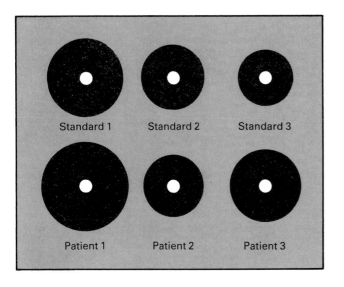

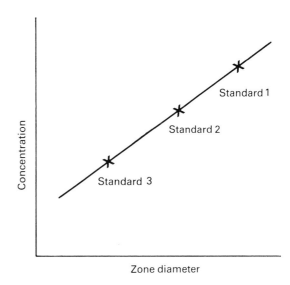

Immunochemical measurement of complement components

These tests depend on the use of specific antisera to individual complement components. C3, C4, C1q, and factor B are most commonly measured.

The most common method of quantitation is *radial immunodiffusion* which depends on the ability of antibody to precipitate its specific antigen in gel. Antibody, for example anti-C3, is incorporated into agar gel on a slide or Petri dish. Wells are cut in this gel and filled with precisely measured volumes of the patient's serum for testing. As antigen (i.e. the patient's C3) diffuses out of the well, it forms a ring of precipitation with the antibody. The greater the concentration of antigen in the patient's serum, the larger the ring diameter. By comparison with zones produced by standards of known concentration, one can calculate the amount of antigen in the patient's serum.

However, for the screening of large numbers of samples, a rapid automated method is now available—*nephelometry*. In this technique, diluted antiserum is mixed with diluted sample and incubated for a few minutes, after which light scattering by the small antigen–antibody aggregates is read and compared with the standard antigen solutions.

In practice C3 and C4 estimation combined with a CH50 titre for overall complement activity are the most frequently used tests for the routine investigation of complement.

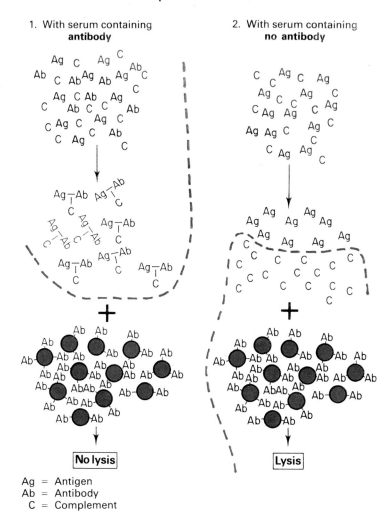

Complement fixation test

1. With serum containing **antibody**

2. With serum containing **no antibody**

Ag = Antigen
Ab = Antibody
C = Complement

Complement fixation tests

Complement fixation tests play no role in the clinical investigation of an abnormal complement system. They are, however, useful tools in the laboratory as serological tests for the detection of antibody.

The principle of the test is first to allow the antigen–antibody system under investigation (e.g. bacterial suspension and patient's serum containing antibody) to interact at 37 °C in the presence of a known amount of complement. Secondly, when this reaction has taken place an indicator system consisting of sheep red blood cells coated (i.e. 'sensitized') with antibody to sheep red cells is added. If the complement was not used up (i.e. 'fixed') in the first stage, the red cells are lysed, i.e. the test is *negative*—no specific antibody is present in the patient's serum. Failure of the cells to lyse indicates that complement has been fixed in the first reaction and indicates a *positive* result.

The test has its widest clinical application in microbiology and in the diagnosis of infectious diseases.

Acute phase reactants

For many years, it has been known that a variety of conditions are associated with an increased synthesis of certain proteins. Measurement of these proteins can indicate in a non-specific way whether an inflammatory condition is resolving.

Two investigations to measure the level of these proteins are commonly employed:
1. ESR (erythrocyte sedimentation rate).
2. CRP (C-reactive protein).

> **Some conditions associated with acute phase reactants**
>
> Infectious disease
> Inflammatory processes,
>   e.g. autoimmune disease
> Malignancy
> Plasmacytomas,
>   e.g. multiple myeloma
> Elderly patients
> Pregnancy

ESR

Red blood corpuscles sediment more rapidly when acute phase proteins are present in the patient's plasma.

Two methods—Westergren or Wintrobe—are used for the measurement of ESR. Both involve pipetting unclotted blood into a narrow calibrated tube and allowing the red cells to settle. Measurement is made after one hour.

> **Normal ESR values**
>
> Men   0–10 mm in first hour
> Women   0–15 mm in first hour

CRP

C-reactive protein is so named because by coincidence, it is capable of precipitating with the pneumococcal cell wall polysaccharide (Group C). This protein is present in extremely low concentrations in the normal healthy individual but its level increases to high levels very rapidly at the start of an inflammatory reaction within the body.

CRP can be quantitated by radial immunodiffusion in a similar manner to complement components.

> **Main difference between CRP and ESR**
>
> When tissue injury or infection occurs CRP rises earlier than ESR
>
> and
>
> When recovery occurs it tends to fall faster

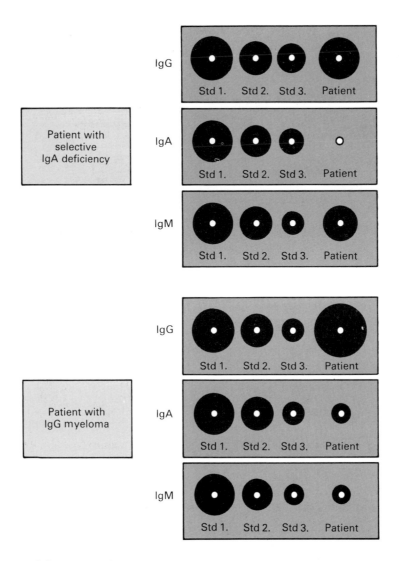

Tests of humoral immunity
Immunoglobulin estimation

Generally when immunoglobulin estimation is requested routinely IgG, IgA and IgM only are measured, using the technique of *radial immunodiffusion* or *nephelometry* previously described for the measurement of complement components.

IgD is measured by a similar technique, but since the function of this immunoglobulin is largely unknown, its measurement is seldom requested except in the rare instance where an IgD myeloma is suspected.

IgE estimation is performed by an entirely different technique of radioimmunoassay and should be requested separately.

The measurement of total immunoglobulins is useful in a limited number of immunological conditions such as immunodeficiency, myeloma, in some liver and autoimmune diseases, and in the monitoring of gammaglobulin therapy in a patient who has proven agammaglobulinaemia.

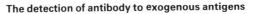

The detection of antibody to exogenous antigens

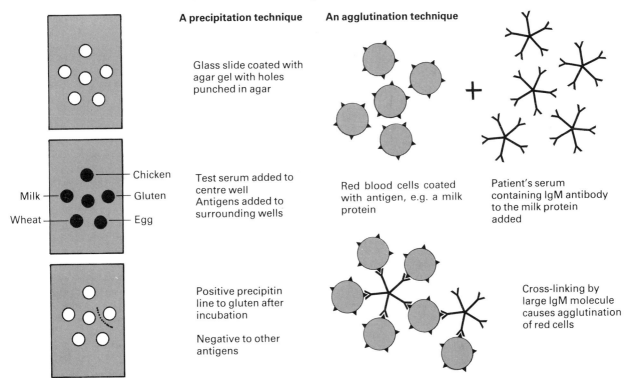

A precipitation technique

Glass slide coated with agar gel with holes punched in agar

Test serum added to centre well
Antigens added to surrounding wells

Milk — Chicken
Gluten
Wheat — Egg

Positive precipitin line to gluten after incubation

Negative to other antigens

An agglutination technique

Red blood cells coated with antigen, e.g. a milk protein

Patient's serum containing IgM antibody to the milk protein added

Cross-linking by large IgM molecule causes agglutination of red cells

The detection of specific antibodies

The detection of specific antibody levels has been used for many years by bacteriologists and virologists in the diagnosis of infectious diseases. In fact many of these investigations are historically designated as microbiological investigations and are not performed routinely in the clinical immunology laboratory. Examples of such investigations are the Widal test for typhoid and paratyphoid, the Wasserman reaction for syphilis, and the Paul-Bunnel test for glandular fever. Microbiology departments have therefore for many years been making use of precipitation, agglutination, complement fixation and, more recently, radioimmunoassay (RIA) and enzyme-linked immunosorbent assay (ELISA)—all techniques that are the basic tools of the immunologist.

Haematologists also for many years have made use of immunological techniques in blood transfusion and in the investigation of haemolytic anaemias. Detection of some specific antibodies, however, is performed in the clinical immunology laboratory.

The detection of antibody to exogenous antigens

Sometimes the presence of high levels of antibody of IgG, IgA, or IgM classes may be associated with certain conditions. For example, children with *coeliac disease* almost always have circulating antibody to *gluten* (a protein constituent of wheat). This can be detected by a precipitation technique.

Milk allergy also may be associated with high levels of antibody to various milk proteins and this can be detected by a haemagglutination technique.

The presence of circulating antibody does not necessarily imply that an immune reaction is the cause of the patient's symptoms. For example, almost all bottle-fed children have high circulating antibodies to cow's milk protein, but this generally reflects a normal response to a large antigenic load crossing the gut mucosa. One must exercise caution when interpreting the results of positive antibody to exogenous antigen.

Another disease in which the detection of specific antibodies can help in diagnosis is extrinsic allergic alveolitis, for example farmer's lung, as almost all of these patients have high levels of precipitating IgG antibody to the microorganisms found in mouldy hay. These antibodies can be detected by RIA or ELISA technique. However, it should be remembered that some exposed individuals can have demonstrable antibody levels but be asymptomatic.

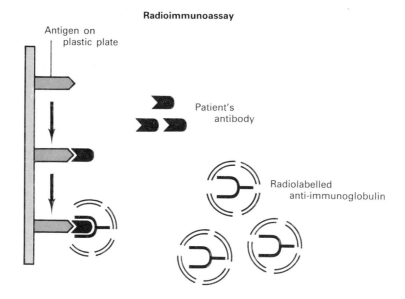

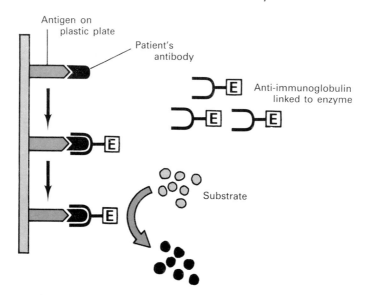

Radioimmunoassay (RIA) and enzyme-linked immunosorbent assay (ELISA)

These techniques are now widely used for measuring specific antibodies. They are both extremely sensitive and large numbers of tests can be performed in a relatively short time.

In both these techniques, the antigen, e.g. milk, is attached to a solid phase such as a plastic plate and the patient's serum is then added and incubated to allow any milk-specific antibodies present to bind to the antigen.

In RIA, radiolabelled anti-immunoglobulin is then added. This binds to the plastic plate via the patient's specific antibody. The radioactivity bound to the plate is then counted, the higher the counts indicating the greater the amount of specific antibody.

In ELISA, instead of being radiolabelled, the anti-immunoglobulin is coupled to an enzyme. It binds to the patient's antibody and a colourless substrate is then added. This is acted on by the enzyme to produce a coloured end-product. The amount of test antibody is measured by assessing the depth of colour change.

One advantage of ELISA over RIA is that it is safer, in that it does not involve the handling of potentially dangerous radioactive material.

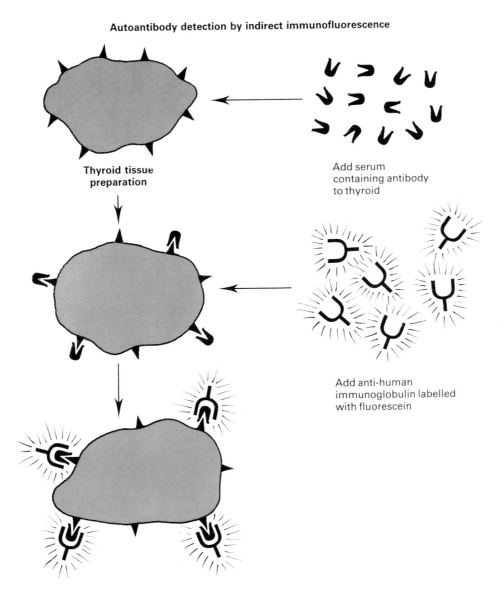

Autoantibody detection by indirect immunofluorescence

Thyroid tissue
preparation

Add serum
containing antibody
to thyroid

Add anti-human
immunoglobulin labelled
with fluorescein

The detection of autoantibodies

Indirect immunofluorescence is the technique most commonly used for the detection of autoantibodies against tissue antigens. This involves the application of the patient's serum, which is thought, for example, to contain thyroid autoantibodies, on to thyroid tissue placed on a slide. After allowing time for binding of antibody to antigen, the tissue is washed thoroughly. A solution of anti-human immunoglobulin which has been labelled with fluorescein is then added to the system. If the patient's serum is positive for thyroid antibody, fluorescence of the tissues will be seen microscopically. If the serum does not contain thyroid antibody there will be no fluorescence.

Similar techniques are used for detecting antibody to smooth muscle, nuclei, mitochondria, and other tissue constituents.

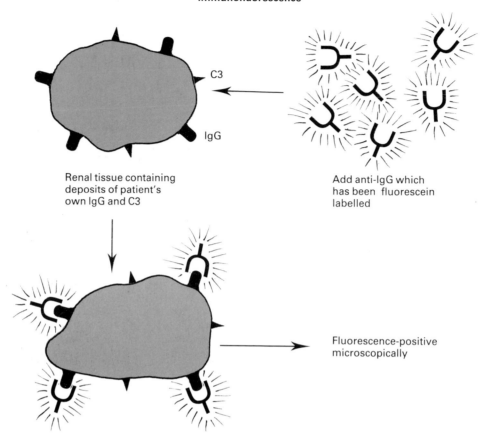

Detection of antibody and complement in tissue biopsy using direct immunofluorescence

C3

IgG

Renal tissue containing
deposits of patient's
own IgG and C3

Add anti-IgG which
has been fluorescein
labelled

Fluorescence-positive
microscopically

C3 deposits can be detected in a similar way using antiserum
to C3

The detection of antibody and complement in tissue biopsies

Some conditions can be diagnosed or classified by taking a biopsy of the tissue in question and using a *direct immunofluorescent antibody technique* to detect tissue deposits of the various classes of immunoglobulin and/or complement.

This, for example, is useful in the classification of nephritis due to either immune complex disease or to the presence of an autoantibody to the renal basement membrane. It is also made use of in the diagnosis of some skin conditions.

Positive control   **Negative control**   **Test serum**

+

R.A. latex antigen

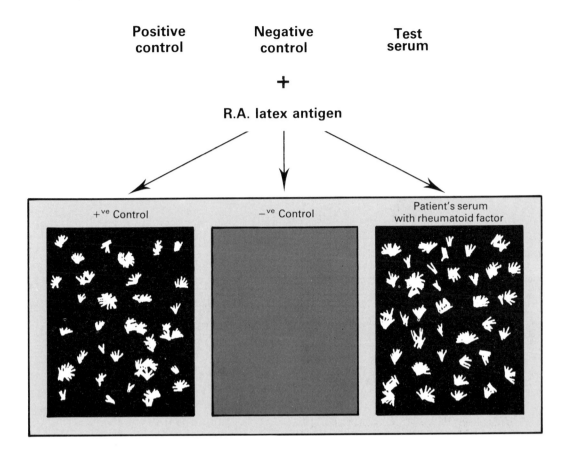

Rheumatoid factor

Rheumatoid factor is an IgM antibody directed against the patient's own IgG molecules. As it is frequently present in patients with *rheumatoid arthritis*, its detection is diagnostically useful, although its role in the disease process in this condition is more doubtful.

The presence of rheumatoid factor can be detected by a *latex agglutination test*. In this test latex particles are coated with human IgG and are mixed with the patient's own serum on a clean glass slide. If rheumatoid factor is present, the particles will be agglutinated within 1–2 minutes.

Some IgE terminology

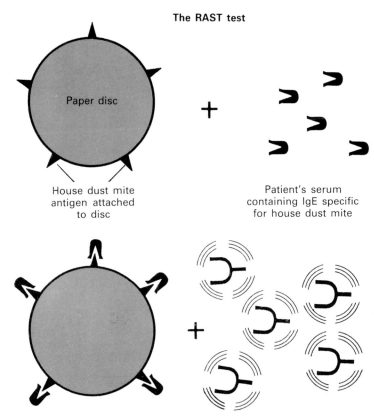

The RAST test

<table>
<tr><td>

PRIST*
Paper radioimmunosorbent technique

measures

Total IgE

</td></tr>
</table>

<table>
<tr><td>

RAST*
Radio allergosorbent technique

measures

Specific IgE

</td></tr>
</table>

Paper disc

House dust mite
antigen attached
to disc

+

Patient's serum
containing IgE specific
for house dust mite

+

Radiolabelled
anti-IgE which binds
to paper disc via patient's IgE

After washing disc, count bound
radioactivity and calculate
specific IgE

Immunoglobulin E estimation

Determination of total serum IgE is generally requested in patients suffering from *atopic* diseases (asthma, eczema, hay fever, suspected food allergy), or helminthic infestations. It is very often elevated in these conditions. It is probably more important to determine which antigens or allergens are responsible for the patient's symptoms.

Since serum levels of total IgE and IgE specific for certain allergens are much lower than IgG, IgA and IgM, a very sensitive technique is required for their measurement. Either a radioimmunoassay (RIA) or an enzyme-linked immunoassay (ELISA) are the methods currently used.

Some of the IgE radioimmunoassay 'jargon' can be rather confusing and so a summary of the current terminology is shown above.

The allergens utilized in the RAST test depend very much on the patient's history; however, a battery of common allergens would be *house dust mite, milk, egg, cat fur, grass pollen, tree pollen.*

RAST estimation to allergens such as horse dander, bee venom, and penicillin would normally be done only in patients giving a possible history of such allergy. A very high proportion of atopic patients have very elevated specific IgE levels to house dust mite, grass pollen, or cat fur, and it is likely that most adult atopic patients could be detected by assaying IgE to these 3 allergens.

The pattern in young children, however, is different. IgE antibody to food such as milk and egg is much more common than in the adult or older child.

It should be remembered that IgE estimation is an expensive technique and should generally be requested only when it is considered to be useful in the diagnosis or management of the patient's symptoms.

★ This terminology is now commonly used and orginates from the names of the kits commercially produced by Pharmacia.

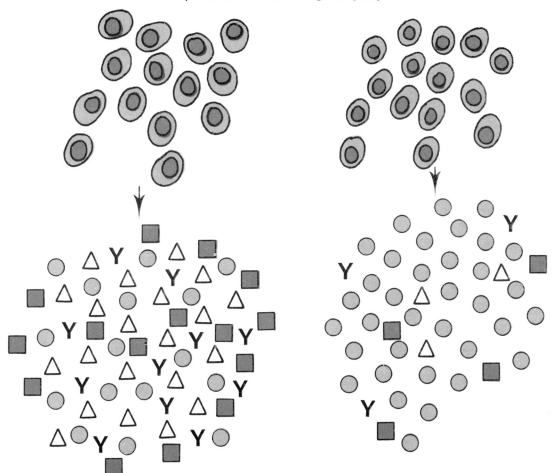

Polyclonal versus monoclonal gammopathy

Polyclonal   i.e. increased amounts of immunoglobulin of various molecular types

Monoclonal   i.e. increased amounts of immunoglobulin of one predominant molecular type

The investigation of multiple myeloma

Suppose that estimation of a patient's immunoglobulins shows an extremely high level of IgG with normal or low levels of the other classes of immunoglobulin. Such an elevation could be polyclonal or monoclonal. It is important to distinguish which, since a monoclonal gammopathy is often a reflection of an underlying malignant process.

The diagram above represents four different types of IgG-producing plasma cells. They have undergone transformation and are actively producing 'clones' of plasma cells.

In a monoclonal gammopathy, a particular cell type predominates, and this is reflected by a large increase in identical immunoglobulin molecules.

The investigations routinely used to distinguish a polyclonal gammopathy from a monoclonal gammopathy are *electrophoresis and immunoelectrophoresis*.

Electrophoresis

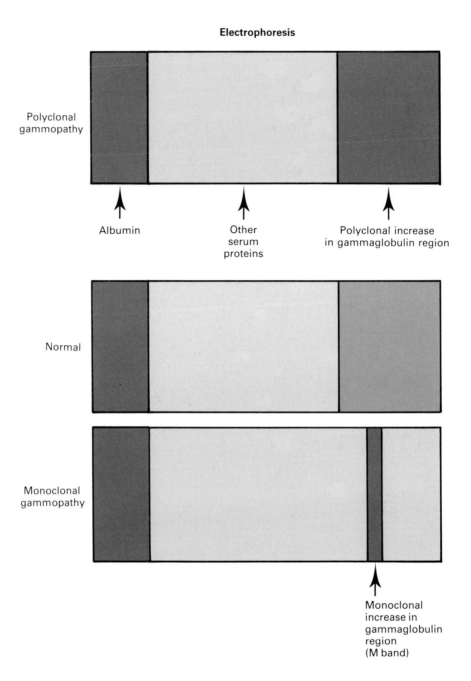

Polyclonal
gammopathy

↑ Albumin

↑ Other
serum
proteins

↑ Polyclonal increase
in gammaglobulin region

Normal

Monoclonal
gammopathy

↑ Monoclonal
increase in
gammaglobulin
region
(M band)

Electrophoresis

This technique involves placing a small sample of serum on a strip of agar. An electric current is then applied in order to separate the components of the serum according to *electrophoretic mobility*. The agar is then stained and various 'bands' are seen corresponding to the different proteins present in the patient's serum.

This technique can distinguish a monoclonal from a polyclonal increase but gives no indication of which immunoglobulin class is responsible. Immunoelectrophoresis or immunofixation is necessary for this.

Immunoelectrophoresis

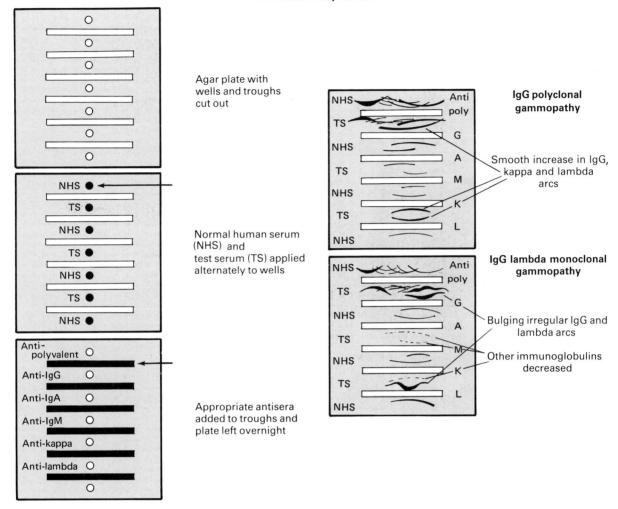

Agar plate with wells and troughs cut out

Normal human serum (NHS) and test serum (TS) applied alternately to wells

Appropriate antisera added to troughs and plate left overnight

IgG polyclonal gammopathy

Smooth increase in IgG, kappa and lambda arcs

IgG lambda monoclonal gammopathy

Bulging irregular IgG and lambda arcs

Other immunoglobulins decreased

Immunoelectrophoresis

Immunoelectrophoresis of serum and urine generally enables identification of the heavy chain and light chain types of a monoclonal gammopathy.

In this technique a glass plate is coated with agar and wells and troughs are cut out.

Normal human serum (NHS) and the test serum (TS) to be examined are placed in alternate wells and an electric current applied across the plate to separate components according to electrophoretic mobility.

The current is then switched off and the troughs are filled with various antisera according to the plan above. The plate is then left for 24 hours for diffusion and precipitation to take place.

Because a monoclonal gammopathy contains identical molecules of the same electrophoretic mobilities,

a 'bump' appears in what should normally be a smooth precipitin arc. This is generally seen in both heavy and light chain arcs. Such a distortion is not present in a polyclonal gammopathy.

Since each immunoglobulin molecule contains one type of light chain only, a monoclonal gammopathy will result in a light chain imbalance because of overproduction of one particular type. When a clone of plasma cells is malignant, abnormal immunoglobulin molecules tend to be produced. In addition to complete molecules, light chains and sometimes heavy chains are produced separately. These 'free' light chains are small and readily appear in the urine as 'Bence-Jones' protein.

Isoelectric focusing

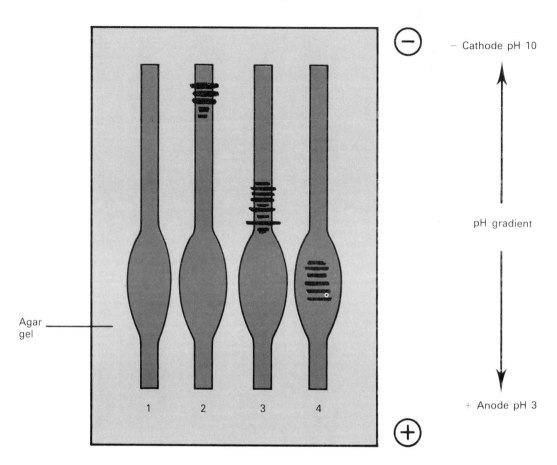

1. Normal human serum showing diffuse staining pattern
2. Serum containing monoclonal IgG
3. Serum containing monoclonal IgA
4. Serum containing monoclonal IgM

Immunofixation and isoelectric focusing

These are other methods which can be used to identify a monoclonal gammopathy. They are more sensitive than immunoelectrophoresis as they detect very small amounts of monoclonal protein.

Immunofixation electrophoresis

In this technique the serum proteins are separated electrophoretically in an agar gel as described previously (p. 164). The gel is then overlayed with a strip of paper which has been soaked in antiserum (e.g. anti-IgG) and incubated for 30 minutes to allow precipitation of the appropriate protein to occur—in this case IgG. The paper is then removed and the gel washed and stained. Any monoclonal protein will stain as a discrete band.

Isoelectric focusing

Isoelectric focusing involves the separation of proteins according to their isoelectric point (basically their pH) rather than their electrophoretic mobility. Each monoclonal protein has a unique pH and is concentrated into a discrete band when separated and stained in a gel. This can be compared with the diffuse staining distribution seen in the polyclonal gammopathies.

The Raji test for circulating immune complexes

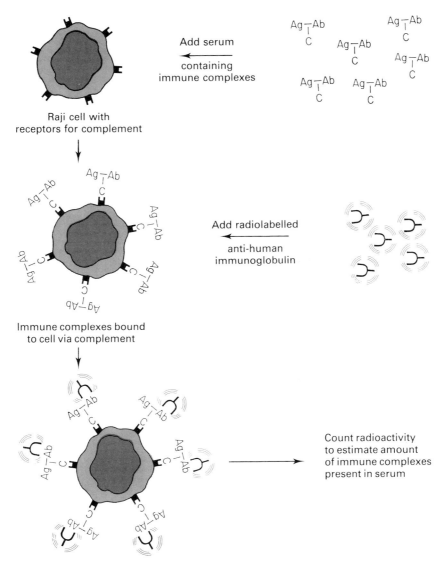

The detection of circulating immune complexes

There are many, many types of investigation documented for the detection of circulating immune complexes. The multitude of techniques available suggests that none is ideal and each has its limitations. Apart from technical difficulties in performing the techniques, the temporary presence of circulating immune complexes is probably a fairly normal event and positive results should therefore be interpreted with caution. Immune complex determination is probably most useful as a research tool in the investigation of immunological disease processes.

One of the techniques utilizing a lymphoma cell line (Raji cell) is illustrated above. Other methods commonly used are:

1. *C1q binding assay*, which depends on the property of immune complexes to bind complement.
2. *Conglutinin binding assay*. Conglutinin is a bovine serum protein which binds to C3 fixed in immune complexes.

Routine lymphocyte assays

	T cells	B cells
Numbers	E Rosettes	Surface immunoglobulin
	Monoclonal antibody to cell surface markers	Serum immunoglobulins Specific antibodies
Function	Delayed hypersensitivity skin testing	Pokeweed mitogen
Blast transformation	Phytohaemagglutinin Concanavalin A	

Tests of cell-mediated immunity

In the investigation of a patient suspected of having a defect in T cell function, *in vivo skin testing* with a battery of common antigens should first be performed. The antigens commonly used are purified protein derivative (PPD), *Candida*, *Trichophyton*, *mumps*, and *streptokinase streptodornase* as previously mentioned. If there is no response to any of these after 48 hours, it is likely that the patient is *anergic*, i.e. suffering from a deficiency of cell-mediated immunity. Lymphocyte function should therefore be investigated *in vitro*.

In vitro lymphocyte assays are routinely used to assess:

1. The *numbers* of T and B lymphocytes.
2. The *function* of T and B lymphocytes.

These tests are performed on living cells separated from a heparinized sample of the patient's blood. It is important that the blood is transported to the laboratory as quickly as possible.

E Rosetting

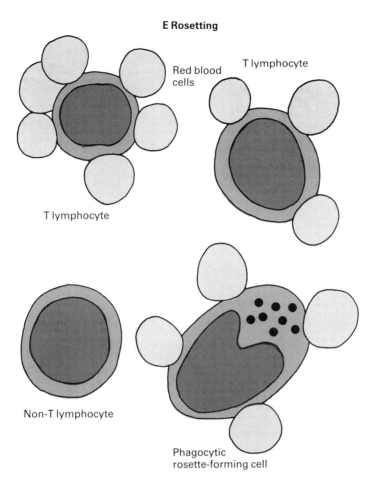

Red blood cells

T lymphocyte

T lymphocyte

Non-T lymphocyte

Phagocytic rosette-forming cell

Quantitation of T and B lymphocytes in the peripheral blood

Enumeration of T and B lymphocytes is necessary in the investigation of primary immunodeficiency states. It is also of use in the diagnosis of secondary immunodeficiency and in the classification of lymphoproliferative disorders (e.g. leukaemias).

T and B lymphocytes are indistinguishable under the microscope. They can, however, be characterized by certain cell *surface markers*. There are a variety of determinants found on the surface of lymphocytes which can be used to identify certain subsets of cells. Some basic methods for T and B cell identification are:

for *T cells*—ability to bind sheep erythrocytes (E) forming an *E rosette*.
for *B cells*—presence of *surface-bound immunoglobulin*.

E rosettes

When normal human peripheral blood lymphocytes are incubated overnight with sheep erythrocytes under certain conditions, approximately 70% will form weak *rosettes* with these cells, i.e. the lymphocytes can be seen in the centre with the sheep red cells closely applied to the surface. These E rosetting cells are mainly *T lymphocytes*.

Monoclonal antibody to cell surface markers

In addition, *monoclonal antibodies* raised against the cell surface markers can be used to determine both total numbers of T cells and T cell subsets, i.e. helper and suppressor T cells. This is done using an *immunofluorescent technique* (see p. 159). These antibodies are highly specific and provide a very sensitive means for detecting cells in suspensions or fixed tissue sections. Monoclonal antibodies can also be used to detect other populations of lymphocytes, i.e. NK (natural killer) cells.

Helper/suppressor cell ratios

Sometimes, results of helper and suppressor cell counts are expressed as a *ratio*, largely because an inverse of the normal ratio was initially thought to be one of the characteristic abnormalities found in patients suffering from AIDS.

These results, however, should be interpreted with caution. *Absolute numbers* of T cell subsets are now considered more informative.

Detection of surface immunoglobulin

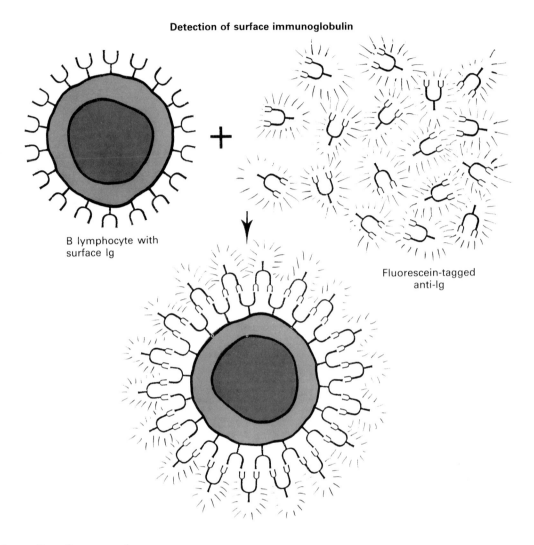

B lymphocyte with
surface Ig

Fluorescein-tagged
anti-Ig

Detection of surface membrane immunoglobulin

B cells can be identified by the presence of immunoglobulin on their surface membrane. This can be detected by *immunofluorescence*. Peripheral blood lymphocyte suspensions are incubated with a solution of anti-human immunoglobulin which has been labelled with fluorescein and then viewed directly with a fluorescence microscope.

Polyspecific antiserum directed against all immunoglobulin classes permits the determination of the entire population of lymphocytes that bear surface immunoglobulin. Antisera produced against specific immunoglubulin determinants, such as single heavy chain or light chain types, allow for the evaluation of subclasses of cells bearing these markers.

B cells also carry on their surface, receptors for the complement component C3 and for the Fc fragment of IgG. These receptors, however, are not specific for B cells (they can be found on macrophages and neutrophils). A rosetting technique using these receptors can be used but it is not as reliable a method for the detection of B cells as the surface immunoglobulin method.

**Lymphocyte transfomration in primary
immunodeficiency states**

Complete suppression: Severe combined
immunodeficiency
Di George's syndrome

No suppression: X-linked
hypogammaglobulinaemia

Partial suppression: Ataxia telangiectasia
Wiskott-Aldrichsyndrome
Chronic mucocutaneous
candidiasis

**Examples of secondary immunodeficiency states
with impaired lymphocyte transformation**

Viral infections	e.g. herpes zoster, measles, AIDS
Other infections	e.g. leprosy
Drugs	e.g. steroids, cytotoxics
Autoimmune diseases	Sjögren's syndrome systemic lupus erythematosus
Others	e.g. Ageing, malnutrition, lymphoid malignancies

Lymphocyte function tests

Transformation responses

Certain substances stimulate small lymphocytes *in vitro* to undergo DNA synthesis accompanied by morphological transformation into large active cells known as *blast cells*. Such responses can be detected by measuring the incorporation of a radioisotope into stimulated cells. This technique gives a quantitative measure of DNA synthesis by the lymphocyte.

This *transformation* occurs *non-specifically* when lymphocytes are exposed to substances called *mitogens*. *Antigens*, however, will transform only *specifically sensitized* lymphocytes.

Mitogens can stimulate both T and B lymphocytes. For example:

Phytohaemagglutinin (PHA) stimulates T cells.
Lipopolysaccharide (LPS) stimulates B cells (in animals only).
Pokeweed mitogen (PWM) stimulates both T and B cells.

Examples of antigens commonly used are *purified protein derivative (PPD)* and *Candida*.

In practice, a patient's lymphocytes are most commonly stimulated with PHA to assess cell-mediated immune status. The mitogen is added and the patient's cells are then cultured in an incubator for three days. Radiolabelled thymidine is then added to the cultures and they are returned to the incubator. The isotope is incorporated into the cells undergoing DNA synthesis and cell division. The contents of each tube are 'harvested' and the amount of radioactivity taken up by each tube is counted. This gives an indication of lymphocyte transformation and therefore the functional activity of the cells.

A microculture technique may also be used. This requires smaller volumes of blood which is important in investigating young children.

In clinical immunology laboratories, B lymphocyte function is usually measured by assessment of serum immunoglobulin levels as these are the end result of B cell differentiation. However, sophisticated techniques for measuring the *in vitro* synthesis of immunoglobulin by stimulated B cells do exist, for specialized cases, e.g. reversed haemolytic plaque assay.

There is a considerable range in the lymphoproliferative response of normal individuals and the degree of reactivity of the same individual varies considerably on repeated testing. It is always necessary, therefore, to test age-matched controls at the same time.

Lymphocyte function tests are essential in the investigation of suspected primary immunodeficiency. In other situations, however, they should be used rather selectively as abnormal results from a single isolated assay are clinically meaningless and do not indicate permanent abnormalities of the patient's cell-mediated immunity.

HLA typing

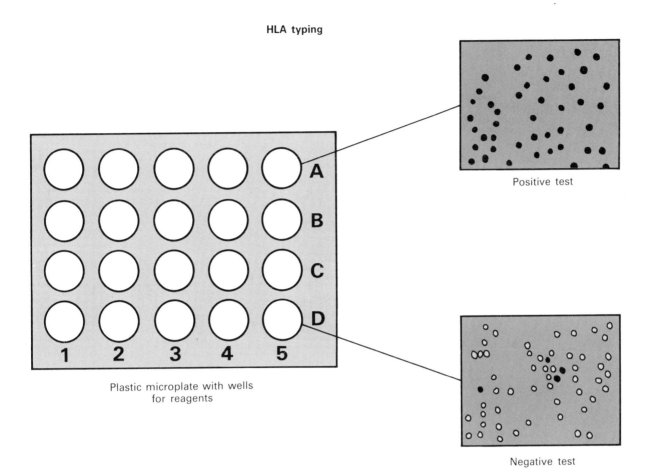

Positive test

Negative test

Plastic microplate with wells
for reagents

30. Investigation of transplantation compatibility

Tissue typing

Tissue typing is the process of identifying the different HLA antigens in a graft and possible recipient in order to obtain a suitable match for transplantation.

The laboratory test most widely used for serological typing for HLA antigens involves the use of sera containing antibodies which are cytotoxic to lymphocytes, i.e. these antibodies can cause cell death when they act upon lymphocytes bearing the specific antigen against which they are directed.

The lymphocytes being typed are incubated in small plastic plates with a battery of antisera to the various HLA antigens. Complement is then added.

If there is an antibody–antigen reaction on the cell surface, the lymphocytes are killed by the complement. A dye is then added and the suspension examined microscopically. Dead lymphocytes take up the dye, while living cells remain clear. The percentage of killed cells in each well is assessed. A strong positive reaction, i.e. the detection of one particular HLA antigen, normally gives 80–100% cell death.

Tissue typing is performed as a microtest in order to conserve valuable antisera and to reduce the number of lymphocytes required for the test when a large battery of antisera is employed.

Mixed lymphocyte reaction

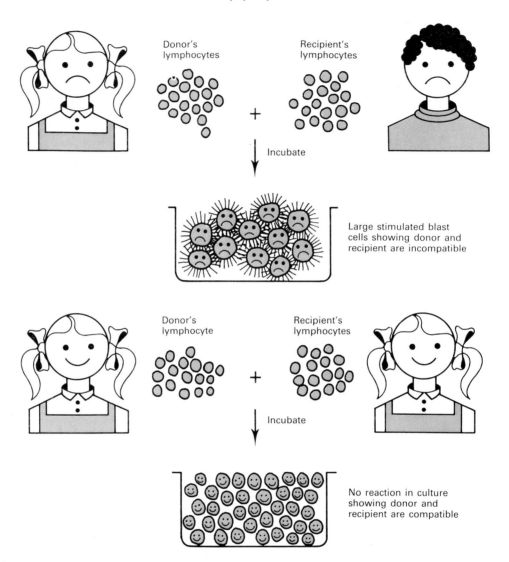

Donor's lymphocytes + Recipient's lymphocytes

Incubate

Large stimulated blast cells showing donor and recipient are incompatible

Donor's lymphocyte + Recipient's lymphocytes

Incubate

No reaction in culture showing donor and recipient are compatible

Mixed lymphocyte reaction (MLR)

The compatibility between recipient and donor in transplantation can also be assessed by MLR.

MLR is not a practical test when organs from cadavers are used because it takes at least 5 days. It is used when live donor transplants are performed and is particularly applicable to bone marrow transplantation.

In MLR, lymphocytes of two individuals are cultured together for several days. In most situations they react against each other, i.e. each stimulates a response in the other, and large DNA-synthesizing blast cells appear. As explained previously the amount of DNA synthesis can be quantitated by measuring the incorporation of a radioisotope into the cells.

Only the lymphocytes of genetically identical twins will not stimulate each other in this way and will show a lack of reaction in the MLR. The greater the HLA incompatibility between recipient and donor the greater the response seen in MLR.

Detection of preformed antibodies

As mentioned previously (p. 81) hyperacute rejection of a graft can be caused by the presence of preformed antibodies in the serum of the recipient induced by previous blood transfusions, pregnancies or a previous transplant.

Preformed antibodies can be detected by testing the recipient's serum against a panel of lymphocytes chosen to include all the known HLA specificities in a test similar to that used for tissue typing.

It should be noted that tissue typing is only feasible in specialized laboratories.

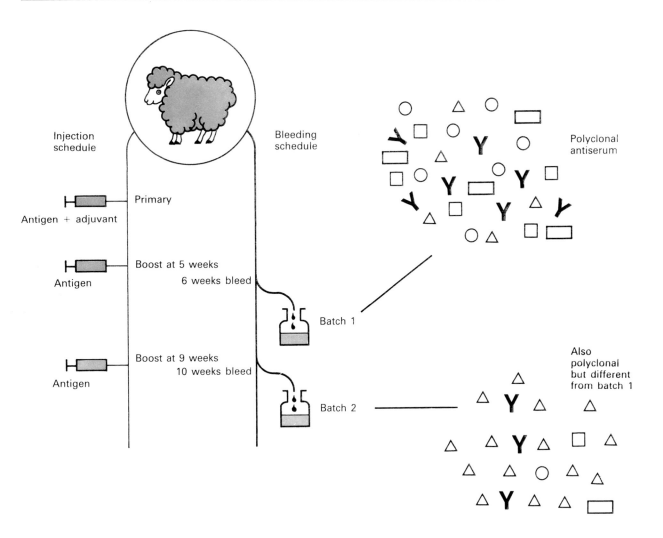

31. Production of conventional antisera

The immunization of an animal with antigen initiates a series of events which result in the entry into the circulation of immunoglobulin specific for the antigen but of different antibody classes and light chain types. These antibodies can be collected and used as antiserum in clinical assays and research. It should be noted that the composition and avidity of antibody in the antiserum will vary from batch to batch.

Production of monoclonal antibody

Immunize mouse with antigen

Myeloma cell culture

Spleen cells

Hybrid cell

Clone antibody-producing hybrid cells

Monoclonal antibody

Monoclonal antibodies

A recent important advance in immunological technology has been the development of procedures for making large amounts of individual antibodies. It is now possible to pass the genetic information in a single antibody-producing cell (which normally does not divide) to fast-growing tumour cells. These *hybrid* cells can be cultured in the laboratory, producing large amounts of *identical* antibody molecules called *monoclonal antibodies*.

The cells both make antibody and survive probably indefinitely in tissue culture because they have inherited these properties from the two different parent cells.

Monoclonal antibodies have two important advan-

tages over conventional antisera, which can vary markedly from batch to batch:

1. They can be produced in unlimited quantity.
2. They have identical specificity.

They are, therefore, potentially very useful in both clinical investigations and research.

For example, they may in the future play a key role in anti-tumour therapy by being able to detect slight differences between tumour and normal cells and so target cytotoxic drugs selectively to the tumour cells.

Currently, monoclonal antibodies to lymphocyte antigens are used diagnostically to identify lymphocyte subpopulations.

Index

g
unology